Core Clinical Skills
OSCEs
in Surgery

D1440497

Ged Byrne MB ChB MD FRCS
Senior Lecturer in Surgical Education and Consultant Surgeon
South Manchester University Hospitals NHS Trust, Manchester, UK

Jim Hill MB ChB FRCS ChM
Consultant GI Surgeon,
Manchester Royal Infirmary, Manchester, UK

Tim Dornan MA BM BCh DM FRCP MHPE
Consultant Physician and Senior Lecturer in Medical Education
Hope Hospital, Salford, Manchester, UK

Paul O'Neill MB ChB BSc(Hons) MD FRCP
Professor of Medical Education and Honorary Consultant
in Geriatric Medicine, University of Manchester, UK

D3010
MED LIB
Ollscoil na hÉireann Leabharlann James Hardiman Gaillimh

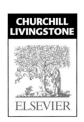

CHURCHILL LIVINGSTONE

ELSEVIER

Edinburgh London New York Oxford Philadelphia St Louis Sydney Toronto 2007

CHURCHILL
LIVINGSTONE
ELSEVIER

© 2007, Elsevier Limited. All rights reserved.

First published 2007
Reprinted 2009

ISBN-13: 9780443071867

British Library Cataloguing in Publication Data
A catalogue record for this book is available from the British Library

Library of Congress Cataloging in Publication Data
A catalog record for this book is available from the Library of Congress

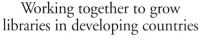

Working together to grow
libraries in developing countries

www.elsevier.com | www.bookaid.org | www.sabre.org

ELSEVIER   BOOK AID International   Sabre Foundation

your source for books,
journals and multimedia
in the health sciences
www.elsevierhealth.com

The
Publisher's
policy is to use
**paper manufactured
from sustainable forests**

Printed in China

Preface

In many medical undergraduate programmes, discipline-specific clinical assessments have been removed in favour of combined. These are designed to assess whether a student has reached the desired competence in a range of clinical skills, which are often not identified as being firmly linked to a specific clinical discipline. Undoubtedly variations exist not only in the knowledge required by specialists in specific disciplines, but also in their styles of information gathering, cognitive thought processes and professional relationships. The traditional general medicine-/general surgery-based clinical curricula of many medical schools has now been replaced by integrated courses, which focus on self-directed student learning. Surgery remains a core activity for doctors throughout the world and its impact is unlikely to diminish in the foreseeable future. The disadvantage of down-playing the place of surgery and surgical education in many undergraduate curricula creates a significant risk that students may not grasp that, at times, a surgical approach to a clinical problem may be better for a patient than a medical approach (and vice versa).

In writing the 'Core Clinical Skills for OSCEs in Medicine', Paul and Tim were conscious that they were writing from the perspective of being specialist physicians. Hence, the emphasis of the book was the way that physicians approach particular clinical skills and what a physician-examiner might expect from students at particular OSCE stations. They were pleased with the generally positive feedback to the book by students and clinical teachers alike and that it has apparently helped students in preparing for high stakes assessments. Nevertheless, they were conscious that emphasis on internal medicine has the disadvantage of not providing guidance as to how you might acquire and demonstrate clinical expertise in other, equally important, disciplines. 'Core Clinical Skills for OSCEs in Surgery' is intended to redress this balance and help you in learning how best to approach a clinical problem from a surgical perspective. Our intention is to provide you with the insight into how a surgeon might manage a particular problem and consequently how you should prepare yourself for an OSCE that might entirely (or in part) consist of 'surgical' OSCE stations. (Many postgraduate examinations in surgery have now moved to an OSCE format.) Some of the stations in the book could easily be found in a 'medicine' OSCE (or book), but here we present them from the perspective of both a student seeking to demonstrate well developed surgical skills within an OSCE setting and a specialist surgical examiner.

Ged Byrne
Jim Hill
Tim Dornan
Paul O'Neill

Acknowledgement

We would like to acknowledge all those who contributed to the final production of this book. We would particularly like to thank Martin, Andy and Nigel for their specialist help, Julie and Alex for their meticulous and painstaking proof-reading, Marian and Julia for their inspiration as skills tutors, Kathy for her administrative patience and skill and the clinical undergraduate medical students in Manchester who continue to inspire us as teachers.

Contents

CHAPTER 1   **Introduction**   1

CHAPTER 2   **The OSCE**   7

CHAPTER 3   **The surgical history**   21

History of breast lump	26
History of dysphagia	34
Presenting a history of dysphagia	38
Abdominal pain: long station	40
Abdominal pain: 5-minute station	46
Rectal bleeding	50
Presenting a history of rectal bleeding	53
History of a lump in the neck	56
Upper GI bleeding	59
Altered bowel habit	61
Painless jaundice	64
Painful leg (vascular)	68
Painful limb (orthopaedic)	73
Back pain	80

CHAPTER 4   **Examination skills**   85

Rectum	92
Skin lump	97
Legs (vascular arterial)	101
Legs (venous)	104
Male genitalia	107

Contents

Neck 111

Abdomen 117

Lymph nodes 127

Breast 131

Groin 136

Hip 143

Knee 148

Ear, nose and throat (deafness) 152

Ear, nose and throat (oral cavity) 156

CHAPTER 5 **Interpretation skills** 159

Endoscopic image 161

Raised serum amylase 164

Chest radiograph 168

Abdominal radiograph 171

Post-operative pyrexia 174

CHAPTER 6 **Procedure skills** 177

Urethral catheterisation 179

Insertion of a chest drain 186

Managing a superficial open wound 190

CHAPTER 7 **Communication skills** 195

Explain the results of an arteriogram 198

Informed consent 202

Communicating with an anaesthetist 209

Index 215

Stations by System

Cardiovascular

Painful leg (vascular)	68
Legs (vascular arterial)	101
Legs (venous)	104
Explain the results of an arteriogram	198

Respiratory

Insertion of a chest drain	186

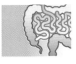

Gastrointestinal

History of dysphagia	34
Presenting a history of dysphagia	38
Abdominal pain: long station	40
Abdominal pain: 5-minute station	46
Rectal bleeding	50
Presenting a history of rectal bleeding	53
History of a lump in the neck	56
Upper GI bleeding	59
Altered bowel habit	61
Painless jaundice	64
Rectum	92
Neck	111
Abdomen	117
Groin	136
Endoscopic image	161
Raised serum amylase	164

Chest radiograph 168

Abdominal radiograph 171

Post-operative pyrexia 174

Genitourinary

Male genitalia 107

Urethral catheterisation 179

Neurological

Ear, nose and throat (deafness) 152

Ear, nose and throat (oral cavity) 156

Haematological

Lymph nodes 127

Locomotor

Painful limb (orthopaedic) 73

Back pain 80

Hip 143

Knee 148

General

History of breast lump 26

Skin lump 97

Breast 131

Managing a superficial open wound 190

Informed consent 202

Communicating with an anaesthetist 209

Introduction

This book has been written as a companion to 'Core Clinical Skills for OSCEs in Medicine' by Paul O'Neill and Tim Dornan. When first published in 2000, there were few if any books specifically aimed at this form of examination in undergraduate medicine. The continuing popularity of 'Core clinical skills' demonstrates the perceived need by medical students for guidance not only in the specific techniques required for an increasingly popular examination format but also the movement towards 'competence-based' assessment within the curricula of medical schools. In addition, Objective Structured Clinical Examinations (OSCEs) are becoming increasingly popular for the assessment of postgraduate doctors. The OSCE was described by Harden and his colleagues in 1975[1] and he later described the OSCE as "an approach to the assessment of clinical competence in which the components of competence are assessed in a planned or structured way with attention being paid to the objectivity of the examination".

Although this book focuses on the experiences of surgeons rather than those of other specialities, you will have probably bought this book because you are shortly going to face a series of OSCEs and you will want to:

* Understand what an OSCE is
* Understand the likely format
* Get to know how to handle OSCE stations and examiners
* Get into the mind of the OSCE examiner so you can perform to a high standard
* Get as many examples of typical OSCE stations as you can
* Get hints and tips for skills and revision techniques specific to OSCEs.

These primary aims are common to all specialities and will be covered in this book. However, because you have bought a book specific to surgical OSCE technique, you may also want to:

* Understand the differences in clinical approach that surgeons adopt
* Alleviate any specific fears you may have in tackling a surgical problem
* Enjoy surgery and wish to excel
* Use the book as you are approaching a surgical postgraduate examination which utilises OSCEs as an examination technique.

We hope that this book will go a long way to achieving these primary goals.

Is surgery different from any other speciality?

Any student who spends time in a clinical environment will know that any two specialists will have slightly differing approaches to the practice of medicine. Communication skills, professional attitudes, teaching style and even diagnostic skill varies from consultant to consultant. There are many reasons for this

---

[1] Harden RM, Stevenson M, Downie WW, Wilson GM. Assessment of Clinical Competence using Objective Structured Examination. BMJ 1975 Feb 22;447–51

including personality type, past experience, length of training and the role models they have encountered during their training. Surgeons will have a different experience of clinical medicine from their non-surgical colleagues. Therefore it is not surprising that, when surgeons are involved in delivering assessments to students, their approach to question setting and examining differs from other branches of medicine.

For example, a consultant physician and a consultant surgeon will have a different perspective on patients with abdominal pain based on their past experience. In the UK, most patients with an acute onset of abdominal pain are assessed and initially managed by a surgical team. The reason for this is that a high percentage of these patients, compared to patients with chest pain, will require operative surgical treatment. Thus the priorities for the admitting surgeon of a patient with acute abdominal pain are resuscitation, diagnosis and a rapid determination of the necessity of urgent operative intervention. In addition, because the patient may need an operation, a standard part of the surgical abdominal history is an assessment of fitness for general anaesthesia. In contrast, clinical experience of abdominal pain for a consultant physician is different. Most patients managed by physicians with abdominal pain fall into three categories. Firstly, there are patients who have chronic abdominal symptoms, referred by their primary carers because of a 'failure to thrive' despite conservative treatment. Some of these patients will have chronic inflammatory conditions or slow-growing tumours. The second group are patients who have come through an acute surgical route in whom no 'surgical' diagnosis has been found. Once again, these patients tend to have chronic conditions where the diagnosis may be obscure. Finally there are patients with 'red flag' symptoms such as weight loss and abdominal pain who are referred for further investigation. With many of these patients, definitive diagnosis may be a painstaking process requiring a thorough 'Holistic' history and many complex and symbiotic investigations.

With these factors in mind, it is hardly surprising that, when faced with a patient with abdominal pain, surgeons and physicians may use different thought processes and learned tools in order to arrive at a diagnosis and management plan, even if the diagnosis and management turn out to be the same.

Why have assessments at all?

There are many (sometimes obscure) reasons for assessments. Modern medical curricula attempt to set examinations that are appropriate for the learning objectives set throughout a period of medical training. The examinations that you undertake whilst learning should:

- Demonstrate to the student and teacher that an educational programme is effective at delivering its objectives
- Satisfy the users of healthcare that doctors are competent
- Provide feedback to act as a stimulus for becoming more able.

The last of these points may come as a surprise to most people. Very often examinations can be seen as, at best, a chore and, at worst, a barely surmountable obstacle over which one must climb to progress to the next stage of learning. The truth is, however, that nothing stimulates learning quite as well as an exam. This has been shown in several scientific studies. Figure 1 summarises one such study that showed that students retained only 5% of knowledge provided during a lecture whilst they retained 70% of the knowledge provided during a written examination[2]. There is little doubt therefore that learning is stimulated by assessment.

Competence and/or excellence

The American entrepreneurial coach Dan Sullivan believes that each of us has our own personalised 'Unique Ability'. Each person's Unique Ability is a set of talents and habits that develop over a lifetime and are those things that we get the most passion for and satisfaction from. In these specific habits and skills, we have never-ending energy and enthusiasm as well as natural talent. Whether we realise it or not, each of us, as medical practitioners, is searching for their own Unique Ability. However, in order to get there we have to work through the stages of ignorance and incompetence before progressing to competence and excellence. Eventually the continuum of learning results in our daily lives being spent doing ONLY the things which truly make a difference to our working environment. Considering this concept pictorially (Figure 2), prior to becoming

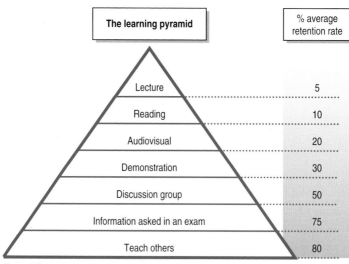

National Training Laboratories, Bethnal, Maine.

Figure 1 The learning pyramid

---

[2] National Training Laboratories, Bethel, Maine, USA

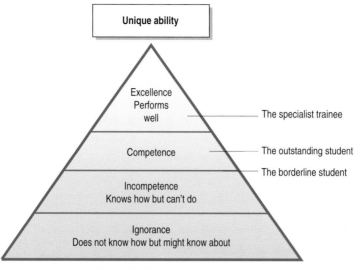

Figure 2 The path to competence

excellent and even unique at a few specific abilities, you will be competent in many things and incompetent in yet more.

An understanding of this continuum of learning is invaluable to success in undergraduate medical examinations. One can draw the following conclusions:

- Learning does not stop following assessment
- No examiner expects excellence but excellence is a bonus (although it doesn't seem like that sometimes!)
- Aiming to be just competent is a dangerous strategy because statistically a 'bad day' is more likely to result in failure for a 'just competent' student than one who is excellent
- Aiming for excellence and not quite reaching it will ensure examination success
- Just because a specific ability or task is not appealing to you, achieving competence in that task is not only achievable but valuable to future learning.

We contend that a good student will not be satisfied by just being competent at a specific task, but will aim at all times for excellence.

The OSCE

What is an OSCE?

The **O**bjective **S**tructured **C**linical **E**xamination was designed to tackle some problems associated with more traditional clinical exams. Perhaps the best-known types of these were the long and short case exams. Typically in these formats, a student was examined by two examiners taking a full history and examination from a patient (the long case) and then taken to see several patients with specific symptoms and signs about whom the student was asked to comment. Variations in examiners and the availability of patients meant that some students had a harder time than others and consequently the reliability of these examinations was poor. OSCEs appear to be a fairer way of measuring clinical ability for three fundamental reasons:

- More skills and abilities can be tested over a specific period of time
- The OSCE relies less on differences in examiners, as many more examiners examine one candidate independently
- Because each individual OSCE station is 'standardised', each candidate can be marked against specific criteria.

Achieving competence?

Clinical competence or performance has been defined as *'the habitual and judicious use of communication, knowledge, technical skills, clinical reasoning, emotions, values, and reflection in daily practice for the benefit of the individual and the community being served'*[1]. If one thinks carefully about this complicated sentence, it sums up the entire nature of the medical undergraduate curriculum that you have worked so hard to master. To put it another way, if, after all your practice and hard work, you are judged by an examiner to be competent at a clinical skill, not only can you perform a particular skill, but also you can integrate and demonstrate your abilities to communicate your knowledge effectively and appropriately, think like a proper clinician and express appropriate emotions in a clinical setting. Clearly this should be a source of great pride to you! It also means, of course, that competence cannot be achieved easily.

Standardised patients, volunteers and anatomical models

One way in which OSCEs differ from traditional long and short case examinations is in the use of simulation. In other words, the exam often tests a student in a 'laboratory' context, rather than at the bedside with a real patient. So, for example, a junior student may be asked to show an examiner that he can go competently through the motions of examining the abdomen of a healthy volunteer without being expected to pick up abnormal signs. Thus, a wide range of skills can be tested without having to recruit patients with specific diseases, and basic procedural competence is tested independently of (and usually at an earlier stage than) competence to detect abnormalities. Simulation allows skills

8

[1] *JAMA* 2002;287:226–35

to be tested that could not be tested on either volunteers or patients. Thus, rectal, vaginal or testicular examinations are tested on anatomical models. The use of 'standardised patients' (volunteers who are trained to take on roles) extends simulation to history and communication skills. In many of the stations in this book, students are asked to take a history, or explain something to a standardised patient. A student may also be asked to break bad news or handle a more difficult problem of interpersonal communication with an actor or other person trained to simulate such situations. In preparing for an OSCE, remember that the emphasis in basic examinations is on simulation and on testing basic procedural competence. Remember also, that there are significant risks in learning all your skills through simulated scenarios. Not all patients present in a 'standardised form' so advanced examinations are likely to test competence with 'real' patients with 'real' symptoms and signs.

The typical OSCE

Examination results that can be duplicated with different examiners at a different time using the same material are said to be 'reliable'. Reliability is a mathematically measurable concept that is used by Examination Boards to demonstrate the 'fairness' of assessments. Generally, overall reliability improves with:

- Lengthening the time taken to examine
- Sampling more broadly across the competencies to be assessed
- Increasing the numbers of examiners.

In an attempt to maximise reliability, most OSCE examinations consist of 15 to 20 'stations'. Each station is independent of the others and tests a different competence. Each station is examined by a different examiner or pair of examiners and normally lasts between 5 and 10 minutes, but can be longer. Thus a group of 20 students undertaking a 25-minute station OSCE would take 100 minutes to complete the examination.

What is being tested

Modern medical curricula use many formats of examination to test students. The most basic assessment, and often easiest to construct, focuses on knowledge. Although knowledge is essential for a firm basis, it acts only as a foundation for higher forms of understanding and behaviours. The complete clinician has learned over a number of years to combine knowledge with a set of acquired skills. He/she uses higher (cognitive) thought processes to purposefully connect knowledge and skills so that he/she can make an appropriate clinical diagnosis and institute an effective management plan.

OSCEs are used to test not only knowledge, but also skills and the application of those skills in clinical practice. Thus most modern curricula use a combination of written assessments and OSCEs to give a comprehensive picture of the student's abilities. It is worth pointing out that different schools utilise

OSCEs in different ways. Some schools may use subject-specific OSCEs (e.g. paediatrics), whilst other schools may examine the whole clinical curriculum using the OSCE format. Thus, it is worth finding out as much as you can about the purpose and format of the OSCE you are facing.

What are examiners looking for?

The introduction of OSCEs with multiple stations has minimised many of the potential biases of examiners. Nevertheless, in order to score well at an individual station, the candidate MUST quickly develop a rapport with the examiner and take care not to antagonise him or her. Although a candidate may be technically competent at the particular skill that the station is testing, the examiner is only human. If a candidate demonstrates an unpleasant attitude, a poor standard of appearance or poor communication skills, an examiner will be predisposed to awarding low marks.

Surgical OSCEs are marked on the same principles as all other OSCEs, i.e.

- A confident approach
- A pace which indicates that you have taken trouble to acquire and consolidate the skill
- Dexterity in performing manual skills
- Good **applied** knowledge
- Comprehensive, clear and considered answers showing that you have thought about the topic before and are not just 'fire-fighting'
- Level-headedness even when the going is tough
- Good communication with both the patient (or simulated patient) and examiner.

However, there are certain characteristics of the surgical 'mindset' which are worth bearing in mind when approaching a surgery-based OSCE station including:

- Being 'slick', i.e. appearing that you have performed the task many hundreds of times before
- Coping with stress in a calm and direct manner
- Being organised in diagnostic and management thought processes (applying the 'surgical sieve': *see below*)
- Giving consideration to the anaesthetic, preoperative and postoperative implications of the task in hand.

Organising your thought processes

Unfortunately, it can be easy for an examiner to believe a competent student to be incompetent. Let's consider an example:

Following a good demonstration of a groin examination, a candidate is asked for the causes of swellings in the groin.

The candidate replies:

" inguinal hernia, femoral hernia... er lymph node and er... hydrocele"

The examiner decides that the candidate is borderline. This may seem a little unfair given that the candidate has managed to recall the four commonest causes of a swelling in the groin in an adult. However, the examiner, who is a general surgeon, considers that the haphazard way that the candidate has presented the causes of groin swelling indicates that the candidate's thought processes are confused. In truth, it may be that the candidate is anxious and tense resulting in a 'blurting out' of the answer. What the examiner is looking for is an organised approach to diagnosis.

He would have preferred an answer that began

"Swellings in the groin can be classified into those that occur congenitally and those that are acquired. In addition, some swellings in the groin are common and some are rare. The commonest acquired swelling in the groin in a male is an inguinal hernia..........."

Classifying conditions, management or complications of surgical procedures is frequently called the 'surgical sieve'. Postgraduate assessment of surgical competence focuses very acutely on a surgeon's ability to use this surgical sieve in making diagnoses and management decisions. Therefore, it is not surprising that surgical examiners are always impressed by students who demonstrate an ability to use this approach.

11

A good revision exercise for surgical conditions is to try to write flow diagrams like those illustrated in Figures 3 and 4. The advantages of thinking in this way include:

- Easier recall under stressful conditions
- More effective learning
- More professional-sounding responses in examinations
- Easier to remember both rare and common conditions.

How are OSCEs marked?

There are two well-used methods employed for marking OSCEs. The first method involves the use of a detailed marking schedule or 'checklist' (Figure 5). This method involves the examiner 'ticking off' components of a competence from a pre-written marks sheet. This system allows the examiner to break down a competence into its parts. A mark is given for each component and then the marks are added to give a total score. One of the problems with such a method is that the examiner can be distracted from the candidate's performance because of constant referral to the marks sheet.

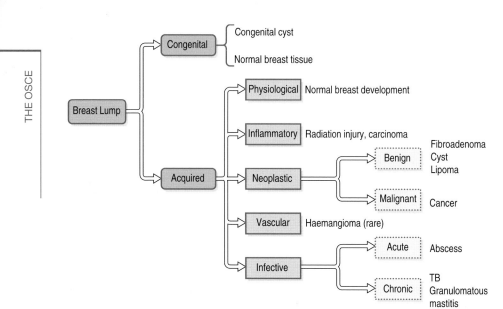

Figure 3 Classification of causes of a breast lump

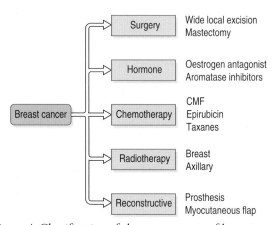

Figure 4 Classification of the management of breast cancer

Some OSCEs employ a 'global' marking scheme. In this method, the examiner is given written criteria (similar to those for the checklist items) and a description of grading for each station. The examiner watches the candidate perform throughout the station and at the end of the station gives him a single grade (mark) based on overall performance. There are obvious pros and cons to both methods of marking, but several research studies have demonstrated a remarkable similarity in marks awarded for OSCE stations irrespective of which examiner or marking scheme is used.

	Satisfactory (1 mark)	Unsatisfactory
Introduction Did the candidate give his/her own name and ask the name of the patient?		
Did the candidate clearly explain the purpose of the meeting?		
Background Did the candidate ascertain what the patient already knew?		
Did the candidate ascertain how much the patient wanted to know?		
Diagnosis Did the candidate clearly explain the diagnosis?		
Defence to battery Did the candidate explain what was going to happen to the patient?		
What will happen on the day of surgery Did the candidate explain what was going to happen on the day of surgery in words that the patient could understand?		
The expected outcome Did the candidate explain the short-term outcome?		
Did the candidate clearly explain the long-term outcome?		
The choices of treatment Did the candidate explain any alternatives to surgery including doing nothing?		
Unexpected complaints Did the candidate explain the possible but unlikely need to change the operative plan during surgery?		
Complications and risk Did the candidate explain the frequency and specifics of the potential risks of surgery?		
Patient's right of refusal Did the candidate make it clear to the patient that the decision is his/hers and that he/she can have time to think about it?		
Check understanding Did the candidate ask the patient to explain back to him/her what was likely to happen?		
Open question to finish Did the candidate ask the patient if there was anything else he/she would like to discuss?		
Record Did the candidate indicate that he/she would go on to complete a consent form with the patient?		
Consent: Repair of inguinal hernia	**Total marks**	**/16**
Overall assessment OUTSTANDING PASS (please circle one)	BORDERLINE	FAIL

Figure 5 Example of a marking schedule for a typical OSCE station. The candidate is asked to obtain informed consent from a man undergoing an operation to correct an inguinal hernia

13

Standard setting in OSCEs

How can an OSCE examination be 'fair'? To achieve 'fairness' a student who can demonstrate a 'minimum acceptable' standard of performance should pass, but a student who falls below this standard should fail. Many traditional university undergraduate courses select a score that they consider acceptable. For example, any student who scores >50% on any examination is considered to be satisfactory whilst those scoring <50% will fail. Although this is a simple way for a standard to be set, many students would consider it to be unfair because one examination set to one cohort of students may be considerably easier than another examination set to a different set of students. An alternative approach is to create a system that measures the relative performance between students in a single group. In this type of standard setting, the students' total scores are recorded and those students whose scores fall into the lower part of the distribution of results will fail (e.g. students scoring less than one or two standard deviations below the mean score for that group). The problem with this type of standard setting ('norm-referencing') is that it makes no allowance for one cohort being better overall than another cohort.

Due to the potential failings of setting standards in the way described above, setters of most OSCE examinations will attempt to define an acceptable *absolute* (criterion referenced) standard. There are many described methods for setting absolute standards but amongst the commonest are:

Angoff[2] method

In Angoff standard setting, a group of experts (e.g. subject specialists) make estimates about how borderline candidates would perform at each OSCE station using a marking checklist. Each member of the panel is asked "What proportion of borderline candidates will be able to successfully pass this checklist item?" After individual rating, the group discusses the items and ratings and explains their reasoning for their estimation and can adjust them. The estimates are then averaged to create a standard (cut-off score). In general, specialists have a tendency to produce high standards.

Borderline method

In this method, the pass mark for an individual station is calculated following the examination. Each examiner gives a candidate a mark based on their total number of checklist items performed correctly and in accordance with the examiner instructions at that station. In addition to this numerical mark, the examiner rates each student as 'outstanding', 'pass', 'borderline', or 'fail'. The mean marks from the stations for all the 'borderline' students is then calculated giving an overall pass mark.

---

[2] Angoff WH. Scales, norms, and equivalent scores. In RL Thorndike (Ed.), Educational Measurement, 2nd Edition, 1971; Washington, DC: American Council on Education.

No standard-setting method is perfect; the obvious conclusion that should be drawn by a student reading these descriptions of standard setting is to make sure that they do not find themselves in the borderline group!

Preparing for an OSCE

Despite every attempt by educational experts, students are always keen to exploit possible shortcuts to achieving high marks in examinations. OSCEs are not an exception to this rule and like most assessments there are exercises that can be performed in the run up to an OSCE that can improve your scores. However, there is no doubt that the competence-based nature of an OSCE demands that a successful student will have done the following long before the examination takes place:

- Practised again and again the core competences that are likely to be examined in the OSCE
- 'Read around' the subjects of OSCE stations in as many subject areas as possible
- Met, taken a history from and examined as many patients as is feasible during their clinical attachments
- Been involved in the emergency care of as many patients as possible
- Practised as often as possible the skills and procedures they are likely to encounter within an OSCE.

There is not, and never will be, a better way of learning in medicine than experience.

During the months and weeks leading up to an OSCE
DO!

- Find a partner who is prepared to practice with you. Ask them to role play a patient with a particular problem (they can use a book as an *aide-memoir* if necessary). Take a history from them, examine them and let them criticise your performing skills
- Study the syllabus on which you are to be examined and pick out those things which are most likely to be examined
- Break down each competence into its component parts
- Read around the subject of each competence and try to imagine how you might answer questions in a logical and classified manner
- Ask the junior and senior doctors on your clinical attachments to observe your performing skills
- Try to arrange for somebody to video you whilst you perform some simple skills: Having done this many times, the authors never cease to be amazed at how shocked students are at seeing themselves perform. Often students can double their scores simply by observing their errors
- If there is a clinical skills tutor where you are studying, try to arrange some practice with them
- Be honest with yourself. Don't keep practising the things that you are already good at, instead focus on those things in which you are incompetent.

DO NOT!

- Believe that you will be able to become competent during the revision period immediately prior to an OSCE
- Practise entirely alone. You will develop bad habits
- Be scared of approaching those people who are already competent and asking them to help.

On the day of the OSCE

DO!

- Get up early, and spend longer than you would normally making yourself look presentable. Make sure your hair is neat and the clothes you are going to wear would be considered appropriate in all clinical situations
- Do a short period of exercise
- Eat breakfast
- Distract yourself from activity that may heighten anxiety
- If your examination is in the afternoon and you are required to be 'quarantined' whilst others are being examined, take a book with you to read and do not get drawn into competitive conversations with fellow students.

DO NOT!

- Find an excuse to go out and party the night before
- Get up and immediately plunge into a revision textbook. The only purpose this will serve is for you to focus on the subjects that probably won't be asked, at the expense of the competences that you will be required to demonstrate
- Panic your fellow students by asking them obscure questions on the way to the examination
- Remember that you have forgotten to have your only suit cleaned.

The OSCE itself

DO!

- Arrive early looking tidy and refreshed
- Introduce yourself in a polite and courteous manner to all patients and simulated patients
- Pause for a few moments between each station (see below)
- When you are speaking to an actual or simulated patient, speak in a clear voice and as far as possible in terms that non-medical people would understand
- Read each task slowly and carefully at least twice
- Explain exactly what you are going to do: even if the object of your task is a plastic model
- If there are facilities available, wash your hands, if not tell the examiner you would wash your hands.

DO NOT!

- Be rude, off hand or make casual jokes
- Physically hurt a patient

- Use multiple closed questions
- Get angry with a patient or an examiner
- Be careless with instruments, sharps or any other equipment
- Be over-confident or over-friendly with the examiner.

YOU ARE AN INDIVIDUAL!

Each of us approaches an examination in a different way. Some people are confident on the outside but very anxious on the inside. Others convince themselves and others that they are useless and get a distinction every time. Preparation for an examination reflects our individual characters. An OSCE is a form of examination that often exaggerates many of these differences and it is essential that candidates tackle any problems they have with the OSCE format before the day of the examination itself. Medical students are often perfectionists. In the course of an OSCE, most people will have at least one bad station; Our perfectionist characters make this an embarrassing experience and it is very easy to take the bad experience at one station into the next station and repeat the poor performance. Most students will develop strategies on their own to stop this happening but some students will find this a problem. If OSCEs pose a particular problem for you, YOU MUST SEEK ADVICE EARLY. Most course directors are familiar with people who find OSCEs particularly traumatic and most medical schools will provide these students with support and strategies to overcome their fears.

ABOUT THIS BOOK

17

Contents

Our aim is make this book complementary to 'Core Clinical Skills for OSCEs in Medicine' (Churchill Livingstone, Elsevier). However, unlike 'OSCEs in Medicine' it is heavily biased towards the surgical specialties. It does not include all the OSCE stations that can arise, but rather attempts to cover the broad principles of examination technique when faced with surgical stations.

Presentation

Like 'OSCEs in Medicine' this book is divided into chapters by the type of skill. Each skill is listed in accordance with its system. There is a tab at the end of each page indicating the type of skill and the relevant system. Table 2.1 lists the contents of the book by system and type of skill. The book is indexed so that you can look up a theme and pick out all the stations where that theme emerges.

Layout of individual stations

At the head of each station, in a similar fashion to 'OSCEs in Medicine' we have used a star rating to indicate its complexity.

- Basic ·
- Intermediate ··
- Advanced ···

Table 2.1 List of stations

Skill	Vascular	Trauma	Gastrointestinal	Urological	Ear, Nose & Throat	Orthopaedic	General
History	The painful leg (vascular		History of dysphagia			The painful limb (orthopaedic)	History of breast lump
			Presenting a history of dysphagia			Back pain	
			Abdominal pain: the long station				
			Abdominal pain 2: the five-minute station				
			Rectal bleeding				
			Presenting a history of rectal bleeding				
			History of a lump in the neck				
			Upper GI bleeding				
			Altered bowel habit				
			Painless jaundice				
Examination	Legs (vascular arterial)		The rectum	Male genital examination	Deafness	The hip	Skin lump
	Legs (venous)		Neck examination		Oral cavity	The knee	The breast
			Abdomen				Lymph nodes
			The groin				

Interpretation
- Endoscopic image
- A raised serum amylase
- Chest radiograph
- Abdominal radiograph
- Post-operative pyrexia
- Urethral catheterisation

Procedure
- Insertion of a chest drain
- Managing a superficial open wound

Communication
- Explain the results of an arteriogram
- Informed consent
- Communication with an anaesthetist

The surgical history

Introduction

Every student 'knows' that 90% of diagnoses can be made on history taking alone. This is a 'truism' that has been passed down from generation to generation. Although the exact percentage of diagnoses made by history taking alone may be open to dispute, its central role in defining disease cannot be overestimated. Moreover, Henry Baron Cohen of Birkenhead, one of Britain's most celebrated and decorated doctors[1] famously stated that THE three tasks of the doctor are "Diagnosis, Diagnosis and Diagnosis". Given the importance of history taking in achieving a diagnosis and the importance of diagnosis in the management of a patient, it is hardly surprising that history taking is the core skill in undergraduate medicine. This section explores the skills of taking and then presenting a surgical history.

Beware the 'type A' surgeon

Many students attending a busy surgical clinic for the first time watch the experienced consultant taking a history and experience a sense of bafflement and dismay. The holistic approach to taking a history appears to be ignored and yet a management decision is often made with supreme confidence. It is true that the pressures of time and the sheer numbers of patients seen in surgical outpatients' clinics have forced surgeons into a system of history taking that does not appear to conform to the structured approach taught methodically in the early clinical years. In addition, surgeons are frequently perceived as having a specific 'personality type', which incorporates a poor concentration span, a short temper, an aggressive approach and an obsession for facts. Although some or all of these features may be true of some surgeons, a closer analysis of the contents of a surgical history taken by a senior surgeon reveals a different story. For the purposes of illustration, let us consider an example of a typical surgical history.

A history taken with experience

Scenario: A 70-year-old woman who retired from the civil service 10 years ago is referred by her GP. The letter attached to the front of her notes reads:

Dear Mr Jones

Thank you for seeing Mrs Smith so quickly. She came to my surgery last week complaining of a lump in the upper outer quadrant of her left breast. The lump was not painful but mildly tender to touch. She has had no nipple discharge or skin changes. I understand that her maternal aunt had breast cancer when

---

[1] Henry Baron Cohen of Birkenhead (1900–1977) Professor of Medicine, The University of Liverpool

she was 80. Mrs Smith has mild angina after walking a mile or so but no other significant past medical or surgical history. On examination, she has a 2 cm hard craggy mass in the upper outer quadrant, which is not fixed to any other structures. There is no palpable axillary lymphadenopathy.

Many thanks for your advice

Kind regards

Yours truly,

Dr R Garibaldi

Setting: A busy breast clinic in a large inner city. Mr Jones is accompanied by a clinical nurse specialist in breast disease and an outpatient nursing assistant into a purpose-built consulting room where the patient and spouse are waiting.

Consultant surgeon (CS): Good afternoon Mrs Smith. My name is Mr Jones, I'm a breast surgeon. Your Doctor has asked me to help out because he feels you have a problem with your breast. Would you like to tell me about it?

Patient (P) *Well Mr Jones, about two weeks ago I was getting a shower and I came across a lump right here (patient points to upper outer quadrant of her left breast)*

Patient spouse (PS) *Is it cancer Doc?*

CS It's a bit difficult to say at the moment. Mrs Smith, tell me a little more about the lump. Is it painful?

P *No.*

CS Can you remember having a lump like this before?

P *No I definitely haven't had a lump like this before.*

CS Have you noticed any changes in the skin over the breast or any changes with your nipple?

P *No nothing like that.*

CS Have you had any breast problems before?

P *I had a bit of mastitis after I had Jimmy but nothing else.*

CS Have you ever had any operations in the past?

P *Only a hysterectomy when I was 44.*

CS Any other illnesses?

P *Nothing serious that I can think of.*

CS	Have you ever had a heart attack?
P	*No.*
CS	Tuberculosis?
P	*No.*
CS	Diabetes?
P	*No.*
CS	High blood pressure?
P	*No.*
CS	Breathing problems.
P	*No.*
CS	Is there any family history of breast disease?
P	*My auntie had a mastectomy when she was 80.*
CS	Nobody else?
P	*No.*
CS	How old were you when you had your last period?
P	*I told you I had a hysterectomy when I was 44.*
CS	Oh yes. Have you got any children?
P	*Yes, Jimmy and Anna.*
CS	And how old are they?
P	*Jimmy is 42 and Anna is 37.*
CS	How old were you when you had your first period?
P	*Blimey! About 14 I think.*
CS	Do you smoke?
P	*I smoked until I was forty but haven't touched one since.*
CS	Are you allergic to anything?
P	*No I don't think so. The cat gives me the sniffles sometimes.*
CS	But you've never had an allergic reaction to anaesthetics, antibiotics or iodine as far as you are aware?
P	*No I don't think so.*
CS	Are you taking any medicines or pills at the moment?
P	*Only the occasional paracetamol for a headache.*
CS	OK, Mrs Smith. Just to recap. You noticed a lump, which is not very painful in the top part of your breast a few days ago. You don't think that this lump has caused you any other problems and you are otherwise fit and well.
P	*Yes that's about it.*
CS	I'm just going to leave the room now. Would you mind slipping your top things off and covering yourself with the blanket. I will be back to examine you in a couple of minutes.

CS leaves room, shutting door behind him.

All of us will be familiar with this sort of scenario. Try timing the above dialogue. It takes about three minutes! Knowing what we do about history taking we instinctively recognise the failings in this history-taking technique:

- The surgeon demonstrates few, if any, of his communication 'skills'
- The 'facts' are all-important
- The patient's feelings are apparently neglected
- The history is almost entirely composed of closed questions.

However, the surgeon will have a very different perspective on the above consultation. Let us try to consider this history from his perspective and take the following into consideration:

1. CS is a consultant surgeon in a busy hospital. He has 15 years' experience in the management of breast diseases as a consultant and deals entirely with women with breast problems.
2. He works in a purpose-built unit with rooms specifically designed for the assessment of women with breast problems.
3. During each year, he is responsible for the assessment and management of some 1750 women with newly diagnosed breast problems, 150 of whom are found to have breast cancer. He has therefore been responsible for the management of some 2250 women with breast cancer in his career to date.
4. He knows through his experience that a 70-year-old woman with the history given to him by the GP has a >95% likelihood of having breast cancer.
5. He has a specialist nurse practitioner accompanying him whose entire role is focused on the emotional support of women diagnosed with breast cancer.
6. He has been given 15-minute appointments, during which time he must take a history, make sure the patient undresses and examine the patient before making a provisional diagnosis and arranging the appropriate diagnostic tests.

Unfortunately, although Mr Jones is acting in a manner that has, to a great degree, been forced upon him by his specific circumstances, his approach cannot be considered appropriate in an ideal clinical world. As a student, you must give yourself the best possible chance of reaching a diagnosis through a careful and structured approach to history taking. Even if we agreed that it is desirable to cut corners, it is impossible to do so if you do not know about the corners in the first place. In the context of an OSCE, a student tackling this scenario in this manner would score poorly. Let's consider a similar scenario within the context of an OSCE.

History of breast lump

Level: *

Setting: Elderly female standardised patient seated in a room with a desk

Time: 10 minutes

Scenario

Examiner (E) Please take a history from this patient. You will be asked to present your history at the next station.

> **Tip**
>
> Read the history as set out BEFORE looking at the learning points and comments. See if you can tell what the candidate has done well and what could be done better.

Response

Student (S) (Makes eye contact, smiles and warmly shakes patient's hand)

S Good morning, my name is Joe. I am a final-year student doctor. I'm very pleased to meet you. Could you tell me your name?

Patient (P) *Andrea Smith.*

S (Arranges chairs so direct eye contact is retained but posture is not confrontational. Smiles.) *I'm sure you know why I'm here but would you mind if I ask you some questions.*

P *Certainly. Fire away.*

S May I ask you your age and occupation?

P *I'm 70 and I used to work in the tax office but I retired over ten years ago.*

S What seems to be the problem?

P *Well about 2 weeks ago I was in the shower and I found a lump right here. (Patient points to upper outer quadrant of her left breast.)*

S That must have been very worrying for you?

P *It was. I showed it to Albert, that's my husband, straight away. I started to cry. I've never had a lump like that before.*

S I understand that that must have been quite a shock to you.

P *Yes it was. I feel a bit braver now though. Whatever will be will be.*

S What happened then?

P *Well Albert could feel it too. He calmed me down and said we should make an appointment to see Dr Garibaldi.*

S Tell me some more about the lump.

P *Well it seemed hard and it didn't really hurt when I touched it. I could move it around with my finger tips. It did not feel like part of me.*

S And what has happened since you first noticed the lump?

P *Nothing really, it seems to have stayed exactly the same to me.*

S Have you noticed anything else about your breast recently?

P *No not really.*

S Have you noticed any changes with your nipple or skin of your breast?

P *No. But to be honest I've never been one for examining myself. I think I was quite lucky to find this lump.*

S So you are worried what this lump may mean?

P *Oh yes. Wouldn't you? You read about so many tragic stories of people with nasty breast lumps.*

S I can certainly understand that you are worried. Let me see if I can find out any more that might help us. Have you had any problems with your breast in the past?

P *No, not really. I had a bit of mastitis after my last child was born but nothing else.*

S How is your health otherwise?

P *I've been so lucky. I've hardly had even a cold. I become a bit breathless now and again after I have walked a mile or two, particularly in winter, but I only need to rest for a minute or two and I get my breath back.*

S Have you ever had any operations in the past?

P *Only a hysterectomy when I was 40.*

S Why was that?

P *I had some changes in my cervix. They took my ovaries out as well. Said I didn't need them! I had terrible hot flushes for a couple of years afterwards.*

S Did you have any other problems after that operation?

P *No. I was home after 4 days and back at work 1 month later.*

S No other serious illnesses that you can remember?

P *No I don't think so.*

S Have you ever had a heart attack?

P *No.*

S Tuberculosis?

P *No.*

S Diabetes?

P *No.*

S High blood pressure?

P *No.*

S Thank you Mrs Smith. I'm now going to ask you some general questions that may help us come up with a solution to your problem. Is there any history of breast disease in the rest of your family?

P *I know that an auntie of mine had a mastectomy when she was about 80.*

S Nobody else?

P *No I don't think so.*

S Do you mind if I ask you some slightly more personal questions?

P *Yes that's fine.*

S You have already told me that you had a hysterectomy and your ovaries removed but can you remember how old you were when you started having periods?

P *I'm not sure exactly but I think I was about 14.*

S Have you got any children?

P *Yes Jimmy and Anna.*

S And how old are they?

P *Jimmy is 42 and Anna is 37.*

S Who do you live with at home?

P *Only Albert, my husband that is.*

S And how is his health?

P *He had a hip replacement 2 years ago but he keeps himself fit. Walks for miles in fact.*

S Do you smoke?

P *No I gave up that vice about 20 years ago and I didn't smoke much before that to be honest: I couldn't afford it.*

S What about alcohol?

P *Oh no. My daughter occasionally gives me a glass of wine at Christmas but I've never really had the taste for it.*

S Do you take hormone replacement therapy?

P *I tried it for a few months after my hysterectomy but it didn't really agree with me so I stopped it.*

S Are you taking any other pills or medicines at the moment?

P *Only the occasional paracetamol for a headache.*

S Have you ever developed an allergy to anything that you know about?

P *Not that I am aware of.*

S You have never had a bad reaction to an anaesthetic, an antibiotic or iodine?

P *No.*

S Okay Mrs Smith, just some final general questions about your health now? Is your weight stable?

P *Yes. I've been nine stone four for as long as I can remember.*

S   Any difficulty in swallowing or abdominal pain?

P   *No.*

S   Are your bowels working OK?

P   *Regular as clockwork.*

S   You told me you occasionally get a bit breathless. Have you had any pains or strange sensations in your chest?

P   *No not that I can remember.*

S   How are your waterworks? Have you noticed any burning when you pass water or are you going more frequently than normal?

P   *No.*

S   And finally, have you had any headaches or blackouts recently?

P   *No definitely not.*

S   Mrs Smith you have been very helpful indeed. I am just going to briefly recap on the important things you have told me. You are 70 years old and you noticed a lump in your left breast about 2 weeks ago. The lump was painless and felt very hard to you and your husband. As far as you are aware you are fit and well and the lump is causing you no other problems.

P   *Yes that's about it.*

S   In order for me to give a proper answer I would like to examine you but are there any questions that you would like to ask me?

P   *No.*

S   Thank you once again (warmly shakes patient's hand). I am sure the doctor will be able to find an answer for you and hopefully sort out your problem. Goodbye.

The differences between these two histories challenge a student in several ways:

1. Why would the consultant's history score lower in an OSCE than the model student answer, given that the consultant clearly knows more about breast disease than the average doctor could ever hope to know?
2. Why does the consultant history just focus on a few bits of a standard history whilst the student is much more comprehensive in his approach?
3. How am I supposed to learn to do well in OSCEs if observing an expert does not show me how to do it properly?

Let's look at each of these issues in turn.

Consultant vs student history

As previously stated, the consultant within a clinic setting has multiple cues and assistance to help him with diagnosis and management, which are not present within the OSCE station. In this scenario they are:

1. A relatively detailed letter from the GP, which has reduced the need for a detailed past medical and surgical history and a review of symptoms.

An 'expert' in the subject is likely to be more familiar with the 'essential' features of a past history through experience.

2. Many years of experience of women with breast disease. This has resulted in a mental 'checklist' including only those bits of information that are absolutely necessary in making a provisional diagnosis prior to examination, investigation and management.

3. The presence of other members of staff with a specific role within the context of a specialist breast clinic. The outpatient nurse's job includes ensuring the environment is appropriate for the initial consultation. The breast clinical nurse specialist is specifically trained to manage the fallout from such a consultation, both in terms of explaining the specifics of the diagnostic process in which the patient is involved and the emotional consequences of such a consultation. So, unlike an OSCE, the environment is specifically prepared for the patient.

4. The consultant will undoubtedly meet the patient again following investigation to discuss the implications of the diagnosis.

This environment is clearly different from that experienced by a student and patient within an OSCE. Not only does the student not have the same cues and support as the consultant, but also the examiner does not EXPECT the same level of experience of breast disease as he or she would of a consultant breast surgeon.

EXPERT VS LEARNER

For most OSCEs, students are expected to reach standards that are similar to those of a newly qualified house-officer. If we consider our learning pyramid once again, students are expected to be competent rather than excellent and thus the examiner is assessing you against a standard of competence and not as though you were an 'expert' in breast disease. This means that the examiner will not automatically presume that if you miss a bit out of your history, that you have done so because you do not consider it to be relevant to that particular patient, rather he will presume that you have simply forgotten to ask the question. Thus the level at which the examination standards are set will determine what you are expected to do within each given scenario. This, of course, means that simply copying someone who has a high level of skill in a particular competence will not necessarily be judged as a good performance within an OSCE setting.

DOING WELL IN AN OSCE

So if all of the above regarding this scenario is correct, then what is the best way of developing your history skills prior to an OSCE? We make the following suggestions:

- Always carry a notebook when observing specialists taking a history. Be sure to jot down any omissions that you observe or any closed questions that you think may have been more appropriate asked in an open fashion.

- Always ask the specialist why he chose to ask a particular question or why he did not ask a question you would routinely ask, but choose the right moment to ask (e.g. after a clinic or at a subsequent teaching session)!
- Observe the environment in which you are learning. Look for non-verbal cues to diagnosis.
- Take time to find out what the other members of the 'diagnostic team' are doing. Follow the clinic nurse or clinical nurse specialist for a time to understand their roles.
- When practising for an OSCE, ask yourself what an examiner would expect of you to get a feel for the standards that are required from you.
- Talk to your clinical partner or members of your peer group about your observations.

About taking notes

The memory is a wonderful thing. There is no doubt that our capacity to remember things is remarkable, yet we live in fear of forgetting. Most students will make copious notes during OSCE history stations particularly if they are required to present their findings in the next station. Although note taking makes us feel secure, there are definite risks associated with it. In our scenario with Mr Jones and Mr Smith, it is quite possible that taking extensive notes would distract and delay you.

- Writing takes time, which is a valuable commodity during an OSCE station.
- Writing requires intermittent loss of eye contact and can distract the examinee from non-verbal cues given by the patient.
- Because we tend to write in the order in which things are said, the resultant page of notes may become disordered when it comes to presenting the history.
- Scribbled writing can be difficult to read.

Try this exercise now. Think of the last patient that you took a history from in a clinical setting. Write a series of headings that you would use in taking a patient history on a sheet of paper, e.g. Name, Occupation, Presenting Complaint, History of Presenting Complaint, Past Medical and Surgical History, Family History, Social History, Drug History and Allergies. See how much of the detail you can fill in for each heading. You will be amazed about how much you can recall about a patient that you only saw once some time ago. If this is true, then it must be possible to remember most of what was said 5 minutes ago in a preceding OSCE station. When you are practising taking and presenting a history, try to do it without notes. See which bits of the history you always remember and see which bits you repeatedly forget. When it comes to writing notes in the OSCE, be as brief as you can, writing down only those things that you repeatedly forget. Some clinicians will only write down drug lists and dates for example. Believe in your own memory's capability!

History of breast lump

GENERAL

| Core skill | Communicating with a patient in order to take a history |

1. The setting

   You and the patient should be comfortably seated at the same level in a way that allows you to face and observe one another without the desk as a barrier between you

2. Non-verbal communication

   No matter how tense you feel, try to establish a friendly, attentive manner. Use a smile and a handshake to establish the relationship; be aware of your posture and gestures during the consultation

3. Introduce yourself, establish the patient's identity and ask permission to take the history

4. Questioning

   - Make as much use as you can of open questions. ONLY use closed questions to clarify what the patient has said, or to obtain pieces of factual information that the patient did not volunteer. Save closed questions until the patient has had a chance to tell their tale

5. Identify and respond to the patient's concerns. Don't ignore a cry for help because you are completely focused on fact finding

6. Summarise periodically and at the end of the interview. By doing this you will reflect the patient's comments back and this will allow you to check your factual information

7. Give the patient time to add information or ask questions

8. Finish by thanking the patient

32

| Core skill | Structuring a history in an OSCE exam |

1. Introductions and consent

2. Identify the main symptoms/problems

3. Use about half your time to obtain a detailed history of those symptoms

4. Use your interpretation of the problem to take a **relevant** past medical, surgical and anaesthetic history, family history, drug and alcohol history, social history and systems review

5. Allow yourself time to think before presenting to the examiner

6. Remember to finish correctly with the patient even if the bell goes!

Core skill　**Applying knowledge while taking a history**

1. Identify the main symptom(s)
2. Obtain information relevant to that symptom; in the case of a pain, clarify its nature, site, radiation, and precipitating and relieving factors
3. Think of different causes of that particular symptom. An 'expert' will frequently tailor their history because a patient reports a specific symptom
3. If a diagnosis seems likely, think of the risk factors predisposing to that disease
4. Think also of diseases that may complicate or be associated with the main problem; for example, ask about stroke and peripheral vascular disease in a patient with abdominal aortic aneurysm
5. Think of the possible effects of the disease on the patient, such as the effect on normal daily living, their job and recreational activities
6. Only ask about completely unrelated symptoms or problems if you have time

History of dysphagia

Level:	*
Setting:	Elderly male standardised patient seated in a room with a desk
Time:	5 minutes

Task

E Please take a history from this patient.

Response

S Good morning, my name is John Temple. I am a third-year medical student. Could you tell me your name?

P *Mr Michael Smith.*

S Thank you, may I take a history from you?

P *Yes.*

S Could you tell me your age?

P *67.*

S Are you still working?

P *No I am a retired bus driver.*

S Could you tell me about the problem that has brought you here today?

P *I have had real trouble swallowing for about 2 months; it seems to be getting worse. I have never had any problem like this before.*

S Can you tell me more about this difficulty?

P *I cannot get things down properly.*

S Which things do you struggle with?

P *The problem seems to be much worse when I eat, it feels like something gets stuck (points to xiphisternum), I seem to be alright drinking.*

S What happens when you eat something more solid?

P *The food gets stuck and sometimes I bring it back up.*

S Are there any foods you now cannot eat or avoid?

P *I have stopped eating some meat, my wife has been trying me with fish.*

S Do you have any sense or feeling where it gets stuck?

P *What do you mean?*

> **Tip**
>
> Read the history as set out BEFORE looking at the learning points and comments. See if you can tell what the candidate has done well and what could be done better

S Some patients can feel where the food gets stuck. It tends to be here (student points to own sternal notch), here (student points to own mid sternum) or here (student points to own xiphisternum).

P *Not exactly but it seems to be lower down rather than at the top.*

S You mentioned that you sometimes bring food back up. Can you tell me how often this happens and what this looks like?

P *It depends what I eat, but it would happen any time I ate some meat. When I bring it back up it looks pretty much the same as when I ate it.*

S Thank you. Have you any pain?

P *No.*

S Have you had any pain in your chest or tummy during the last 2 months during the time you have had difficulty swallowing?

P *No.*

S Has your weight changed?

P *Yes I've lost about 1 stone.*

S Have you had any problems with indigestion or heartburn in the past?

P *No, not really. I take an occasional Rennie's but not very often.*

S How are your bowels working?

P *They're very regular, they always have been.*

S Have you noticed any blood or mucus when you open your bowels?

P *No.*

S Thank you, I have got a clear picture of the problems that you have had with your swallowing. I would like to ask you a few other questions if I may. Have you got any problems with your chest?

P *No, not really.*

S Have you coughed up any blood or phlegm in the last 2 months?

P *No.*

S Do you smoke?

P *No I have never smoked.*

S Have you had any operations on your chest or your abdomen?

P *No I haven't.*

S Would you mind if I just went over that again with you. Can you tell me if I've got everything.

P *Yes.*

S Thank you Mr Smith. As I understand it you are a 67-year-old man who has noticed a difficulty in swallowing which has got worse over the last 2 months. It is more difficult for you to swallow solid food rather than liquids. You have had no other problems except that you have lost about one stone in weight.

P *Yes that's about right.*

S Thank you Mr Smith for you help (student offers hand).

The bell sounds for the end of the station.

Comment

Taking a history from an uncommunicative patient can be off putting. The patient has, however, given clear and precise answers to the questions.

What did the candidate do right?

- Polite at all times despite short answers from patient
- Good use of open questions (although the candidate did resort to some closed questions which were probably unnecessary at times)
- Good structure and order to history
- Good initiation and ending of history
- The candidate offers a summary to the patient.

How might the candidate have improved?

- There is no mention of the patient's feelings or worries as to underlying cause; therefore, the candidate has no opportunity to empathise with the patient's condition
- There is no assessment of past medical and surgical history, which may have been relevant.

Learning points

Dysphagia is often a symptom of serious disease and requires urgent investigation. It is important to establish the length of history and if the symptoms are intermittent, progressive or constant. Sometimes oesophageal obstruction is accompanied by hiccup. The commonest cause of painless dysphagia in an elderly patient is a carcinoma of the oesophagus or gastro-oesophageal junction. This disease is rare before the age of 40 and is particularly common in the Far East and Africa. Men are more commonly affected than women.

The majority of oesophageal cancers are squamous cell carcinomas and most of these occur in the middle third of the oesophagus. Adenocarcinomas are normally associated with 'Barrett's[2]' oesophagus and arise at the distal end of the oesophagus. Dysphagia due to benign stricture can occur even in the absence of a significant history of gastro-oesophageal reflux. There are numerous causes of benign strictures (see Table 3.1), but most are rare.

Extrinsic compression can originate in the neck or chest. Patients can often give an approximate indication whether the obstruction is high, suggesting a cervical or pharyngo-laryngeal problem. In the chest, compression is most commonly due to bronchial carcinoma, hence the need to ask about respiratory symptoms.

[2] Norman Rupert Barrett (1903–1979) Thoracic Surgeon born in Australia who studied medicine and practiced in Britain

---

Box 3.1 The oesophagus

1. A hollow muscular tube
2. 25 cm long
3. Starts at the level of the 6th vertebra
4. Inner circular muscle, outer longitudinal muscle
5. Lined by squamous epithelium
6. Systemic–portal anastomosis at distal end
7. Upper and mid-oesophagus drains to thoracic and cervical nodes
8. Lower oesophagus drains to gastric and celiac nodes

Suggestions for further practice

Although dysphagia is a common focus of examination questions, rationalisation of health services very often results in most patients being investigated in a few specialist units. If you do not have easy access to one of these units, try sketching a history that may be given by an idealised patient with a specific cause of dysphagia.

Box 3.2 Causes of dysphagia

Be familiar with:

- Carcinoma of the oesophagus
- Benign stricture
- External mediastinal masses (e.g. lung cancer)
- Stroke and Parkinson's[3] disease
- Diffuse oesophageal spasm
- Foreign body
- Achalasia (rare but a favourite with examiners because of its unusual symptoms)
- Scleroderma (again rare but patients with scleroderma are used in examinations).

Rare causes (interest only):

- Post-cricoid web
- Hypopharyngeal diverticulum
- Myotonic dystrophy
- Oculopharyngeal muscular dystrophy
- Myasthenia gravis
- Enlarged left atrium or aorta
- Aberrant subclavius muscle.

---

[3] James Parkinson 1755–1824. English Physician who published his "Essay on the Shaking Palsy" in 1812

Presenting a history of dysphagia

Level:	*
Setting:	Single examiner
Time:	5 minutes

Task

E You have just taken a history from a patient with difficulty in swallowing. Please present the history to me.

Response

S Mr Michael Smith is a 67-year-old man who is a retired bus driver. He has a 2-month history of difficulty in swallowing which is gradually getting worse. The dysphagia is principally noticed with solids, so much so that he has stopped eating meat. He vaguely localises the dysphagia to the lower part of his chest. There is no associated pain. He has lost about 1 stone in weight. He has no other gastrointestinal symptoms and his bowels are working normally. He has no associated respiratory symptoms and has never smoked.

Comment

What has the candidate done well?

- Clear concise presentation with good introduction
- Appropriate use of medical terminology
- No unnecessary bits of information, only relevant facts.

Where could the candidate have improved?

It is easy to see from the examiner's perspective how this student may struggle with the next part of the station because this is entirely dependent on the QUALITY of the history taken in the previous station and the student has omitted to ask questions of the patient that the examiner may consider to be relevant. At this time the examiner will attempt to clarify the history by asking related questions such as: Has the patient had any operations before? How does the patient feel about his condition? In addition, a surgical examiner may well be interested to find out if the patient is fit for anaesthesia. The candidate will struggle with any of these questions.

The station continues:

E What is the likely cause of this gentleman's dysphagia?

S Given the history of dysphagia to solids rather than liquids, the associated weight loss and the patient's age, I think that the most likely diagnosis is a stricture in the lower end of the oesophagus, most likely a malignant stricture.

Comment

True mechanical obstruction of the oesophagus due to a tumour will result in a gradual narrowing and a reduction of the elasticity of the oesophagus. Liquids will be able to pass through such an obstruction much easier than a solid bolus of food. With conditions that are associated with oesophageal spasm, liquid often stimulates the spasm (often hot drinks such as tea or coffee) more than a bolus of food.

E What are the other causes of dysphagia?

S Dysphagia can be caused by a mechanical or functional blockage of the oesophagus. The causes of such an obstruction can be congenital or acquired, benign or malignant. In addition they can arise from within the lumen of the oesophagus, within the wall of the oesophagus or can be caused by extrinsic compression.

Note the exact phrasing of the question initially asked by the examiner. The use of the word 'likely' tells the candidate that the examiner wants the student to express a diagnostic opinion. It is, therefore, appropriate to tell the examiner what you think. The second question is generic and requires application of a structured approach, as discussed in Chapter 2.

Core skill   Presenting a history

1. Structure your history clearly and concisely
2. Express it accurately and economically. Concentrate only on RELEVANT negatives
3. Show signs of thought
4. Do not forget to include information that you have elicited from your review of systems which may influence your diagnosis (in this example the importance of respiratory history in determining an extrinsic cause of dysphagia)
5. Specifically refer to previous operations, issues which may pose problems for the patient undergoing general anaesthetic and serious medical problems which may affect management decisions (e.g. diabetes)
6. Report the patient's perceptions and concerns. Is the patient worried about the potential diagnosis and its implications? Does the patient have insight into his/her illness?
7. Offer a diagnosis and suggest what to look for in the examination
8. Offer an investigation and management plan

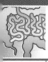

Abdominal pain: long station

GASTROINTESTINAL

Level:	*/**
Setting:	55-year-old patient in a bed
Time:	10 minutes

Comment

The length of time allocated for a given station may tell you a lot about what is expected of you. OSCEs often consist of multiple 5-minute stations, but many merge two stations together if the task is complicated and some allow even more time. Normally the marks available for the station reflect the amount of time allocated for it.

Task

E Mrs Smith is a 55-year-old lady who was admitted through the Accident and Emergency department last night with abdominal pain. You are a foundation trainee (house-officer). Please take a history from her.

Response

S Good morning Mrs Smith, my name is Patrick Holmes I am a third-year junior doctor. May I ask you some questions?

P *Yes.*

40

S Could you tell me about the problem that has brought you into hospital?

P *The pain has been here (briefly points to her abdomen), I've had it on and off for 3 months. It's been very severe when it has come on.*

Comment

Although it is usually sensible to ask an open question first, the patient will give you a variable amount of information and often not in the order you would exactly like it. Make sure you have got a clear answer to each question and prepare to be flexible about the order of questions you ask.

S Can you just show me with one finger where the pain is?

P *Yes.*

(Patient uses palm of hand to indicate pain at the top of her abdomen)

S Was the pain over part of or your entire upper abdomen?

P *It was mainly in the middle and the right side.*

S You said you have had the pain for 3 months, can you tell me what has happened to the pain since it started?

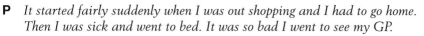

P   *It started fairly suddenly when I was out shopping and I had to go home. Then I was sick and went to bed. It was so bad I went to see my GP.*

S   How long did that first attack last?

P   *About 3 days. The GP gave me some painkillers for it.*

S   How often are you getting the pain?

P   *I have had it three times since the first episode.*

S   You said that the pain was severe, how bad was it compared to other pains that you have had before?

P   *It was the worst pain I can remember. It was worse than giving birth!*

S   Can you describe the pain?

P   *It was mostly a gripping pain, but sometimes it was stabbing.*

S   When the pain was severe, did it make you want to keep still or move around?

P   *When it was bad I couldn't get comfortable.*

S   Did the pain move anywhere?

P   *How do you mean?*

S   Did it go to the lower part of your abdomen?

P   *No.*

S   Did it go through to your back?

P   *Yes, it did.*

S   Did it go to your shoulder (student points to patient's right shoulder)?

P   *Not that I remember.*

S   Did anything make the pain better or worse?

P   *No.*

S   Is there anything you can think of that brought the pain on?

P   *No, not really.*

S   How did you feel between attacks?

P   *Yes I felt fine, I seemed to go back to normal.*

S   Tell me about the next attack you had?

P   *It started about 3 days ago and lasted until this morning. It felt almost the same as the last one, but may have been a little worse.*

S   And what was it about this attack that brought you into hospital.

P   *To be honest, the attacks seem to be getting more severe. I just couldn't bare the pain yesterday so my husband called an ambulance.*

S   That must be very worrying for you.

P   *Yes I am quite scared. I have had some mild tummy pains in the past but the fact that this pain is so bad and keeps getting worse makes me worry that there is something serious going on.*

S   I can understand how worrying that must be for you. Hopefully we will be able to find out what the cause of your pain is and make it better.

GASTROINTESTINAL

41

P *I hope so (patient smiles).*

S Apart from the pain, did you have any other symptoms or problems?

P *How do you mean?*

S Did you feel sick and were you sick/vomiting?

P *Yes I was sick a few times when the pain was really bad.*

S Has your weight changed recently?

P *I don't think so; I may have lost a couple of pounds.*

S Have you noticed your skin going yellow in the last few months?

P *No.*

S Have you been into hospital before?

P *No.*

S How you have your bowels been recently?

P *They have become a little more stubborn than they used to be over the last 3 months.*

S Have you noticed any blood or mucus when you open your bowels?

P *No.*

S How often are you opening your bowels at the moment?

P *Once every 2 or 3 days at the moment.*

S And what used to be normal for you?

P *Once a day in the morning for most of my life.*

S How is your appetite?

P *It's OK except when I get this pain. I just don't feel like eating then.*

S Tell me about your health previously.

P *I had a heart attack when I was 49 and spent 5 days in hospital after it.*

S Has the heart attack left you with any long-lasting difficulties?

P *I get a bit breathless when I walk to the shops. They are about 400 yards away. Sometimes I have to stop to get my breath.*

S Have you had any problems with your heart since that attack?

P *Not really, no.*

S Has anyone ever told you why they think you had the attack in the first place?

P *Apparently high cholesterol runs in the family.*

S Have you had any other serious illnesses?

P *Not that I can remember.*

S Have you ever had any of these illnesses: TB, high blood pressure, diabetes, epilepsy or asthma?

P *No I don't think so.*

S Are you taking any tablets or medicines?

P *Only some tablets for blood pressure and some tablets to lower my cholesterol.*

S Do you know what they are called?

P *I can't remember I'm afraid. Oh and I do take an aspirin once a day.*

S That's OK we can find out later. Do you smoke?

P *No.*

S Have you ever smoked?

P *Well yes. I started smoking when I was about 18 and smoked 20 cigarettes a day until I had my heart attack.*

S How much alcohol do you drink?

P *Almost nothing and I never have done.*

S Do you suffer from any allergies that you know about?

P *Not that I know of.*

S You have never had any strange reactions to anaesthetics, antibiotics or iodine.

P *Not that I can think of.*

Comment

This history is not straightforward. In contrast to history 5, this patient's symptoms are not immediately diagnostic. In addition, there is pre-existing co-morbidity that may affect the risks of this patient during an operation. It is likely that such a station would be set, not just to test the candidate's ability to extract a history of abdominal pain, but also to assess the candidate's ability to judge the patient as a whole. When presenting this history, the examiner will ask about the patient's cardiovascular problems in relation to their risks during surgery.

The student has done very well so far. The history is well structured, comprehensive and thorough. He has tried to ask open questions and occasionally followed these questions up with a more closed approach to elicit a specific symptom. At this point, most of the relevant details have been ascertained. The student has also demonstrated an ability to acknowledge the patient's fears.

43

If you have time, a review of systems is a useful adjunct to the surgical history. The systems review is a series of questions (often closed), which can be used as a 'safety net', reducing the chances of you missing an important symptom that will influence your subsequent patient investigation and management. It is good practice to start with the system that is most relevant to the patient's presenting complaint (in this case the gastrointestinal system) and then work your way through the remaining systems that may be relevant. The systems review has specific importance in the surgical history, because the patient may subsequently require a general anaesthetic. You must also remember:

- The systems review should be an adjunct to your history and should be brief and tailored to the individual patient.
- Don't get bogged down with symptoms that are unlikely to influence your management decisions.

GASTROINTESTINAL

In this case you may want to ask about

Gastrointestinal
> Dysphagia
> Rectal bleeding
> Altered bowel habit

Respiratory
> Shortness of breath
> Orthopnoea
> Cough
> Sputum

Cardiovascular
> Leg pain on walking
> Angina

Neurological
> Blackouts
> Headaches
> Poor balance
> Limb weakness
> Back pain

Genitourinary
> Dysuria

You should be absolutely confident with a common symptom such as abdominal pain. There are lots of questions that must be asked. The skill is to know how to phrase the standard questions to be asked and to be able to synthesise the answers.

Core skill	Abdominal pain

You must ascertain the following from **all** patients with abdominal pain:
Site
Severity
Character
Radiation
Onset
Periodicity
Exacerbating and relieving factors
Associated symptoms

When thinking about the causes of abdominal pain, firstly think of the relevant anatomy at the site of the pain. This is a useful exercise as the site of pain is very often characteristic of specific diseases (e.g. right hypochondrium and gallbladder disease or right iliac fossa and appendicitis).

Then think about the nature of the pain. If it is intermittent and colicky/gripping pain, consider obstruction of a hollow viscus, such as biliary colic, renal colic, small and large bowel obstruction. If the pain is continuous and aching, think of inflammatory or malignant causes. Continuous pain exacerbated by movement is seen with peritoneal irritation; appendicitis, cholecystitis, perforated peptic ulcer, pancreatitis, diverticulitis. Radiation of pain can be particularly helpful and is most likely to require a closed question (e.g. loin pain radiating to the groin/genitalia in renal colic, right upper quadrant pain to the tip of the right scapula in biliary pain, abdominal pain radiating to the shoulder in diaphragmatic irritation, peptic ulcer pain radiates through to the centre of the back, pancreatic pain radiates through to centre of the back, relieved by sitting forwards).

Associated symptoms:

- Upper abdominal pathology is more likely to be associated with upper gastrointestinal symptoms such nausea and vomiting.
- Lower abdominal pathology is more likely to be associated with a change in bowel habit.

Table 3.1 Characteristics of colicky abdominal pain

	Small bowel	**Large bowel**	**Ureteric**	**Biliary**
Site	Peri-umbilical	Lower abdominal	Loin	Right hypochondrium
Radiation	None	None	Groin/penis	Back
Severity	Mild/moderate	Mild/moderate	Severe	Severe
Duration	Peaks last for 30 seconds or so then ease for 15 minutes	Peaks last for several minutes then ease for half an hour	Peaks last for 30 seconds then ease for several minutes	Peaks last for several hours then ease for several days

Suggestions for further practice

Given that the abdomen contains so many different organs, taking a history of abdominal pain is one of the more difficult tasks as a student and takes practice. This is further compounded by the trouble that many patients have in localising symptoms. Many patients on a ward receiving general surgical emergencies will have some abdominal pain and you should take histories from such patients. Do not worry about approaching them as nearly all patients are happy to let you take a history and many will be happy for you to examine them as long as you are gentle.

Try to follow up their case; what investigations have been ordered, what did they show, did the patient require an operation? Often the best way to understand a patient's symptoms is to watch their operation. By doing this it is easier to demystify the clinical anatomy. The observed pathology often tallies beautifully with the symptoms.

Abdominal pain: 5-minute station

Level:	*
Setting:	35-year-old man sat in a chair
Time:	5 minutes

Task

E Please take a history from this patient who was admitted to a surgical assessment ward through the accident and emergency department in the early hours of this morning.

S Good afternoon. My name is John Smith and I am a student doctor. May I ask your name?

P *I'm Fred Jones. Good to meet you.*

S I would like to ask you some questions. Is that OK?

P *Yes sure. How can I help?*

S Would you mind telling me how old you are and what you do for a living.

P *I'm 35 and I work in a foundry on the smelts.*

S What seems to be troubling you at the moment?

P *Well to be honest nothing at the moment but I had a terrible time a few hours ago.*

S Can you tell me what happened?

P *I was working and all of a sudden I got a terrible pain in my stomach. It was agony.*

S That must have been very distressing.

P *Yes, I didn't know what was happening. I was scared stiff. I thought I was going to die or something.*

S Can you tell me more about this pain?

P *Yes it was right here (points to left upper outer quadrant of abdomen). It came on suddenly and then seemed to come and go. It went completely after 2 hours.*

S On a scale of one to ten, with ten being the most amount of pain you could imagine and 1 being no pain, how bad would you say the pain was?

P *A nine and a half I think.*

S Dear me that must have been really awful for you.

P *It was when it happened but it seemed to ease off after a couple of minutes but then it came back with a vengeance about 5 minutes later.*

S How many attacks like that did you have?

P *Oh about ten in all. Each one was just as bad.*

S How would you describe this pain?

P *I don't really know what you mean.*

S Was it sharp or dull or burning?

P *Sharp I'd say, like somebody stabbing me.*

S I know you said that the pain was there (points to left upper outer quadrant of abdomen) but did it seem to go anywhere else?

P *Well that's the weird thing; I could swear it was sending electric shocks into my groin.*

S Did anything seem to make the pain better?

P *Actually if I moved around a lot it seemed to ease a bit and then when I came into casualty they gave me an injection and it disappeared within minutes.*

S Did anything seem to make it worse?

P *Not that I noticed.*

S Thank you Mr Jones, that's very clear. I am now going to ask you some other questions if I may? Have you ever had a pain like this before?

P *No; I would definitely have remembered.*

S I presume working in a foundry is a heavy job. Does it get very hot?

P *Oh yes, it's hard physical work and the furnaces are very warm; I was working on the furnaces today. Sometimes you have to drink gallons of water because you lose it so quick.*

S Did you drink much today?

P *No not really. The water fountain at work was broken so I had to go to the bathroom every time I was thirsty to get a drink.*

S Have you passed water since the pain started?

P *Funnily enough I felt like I wanted to but couldn't whilst the pain was there but I went for a wee just after they gave me that injection.*

S Did you notice anything abnormal about your urine?

P *No, but to be honest I didn't look very hard. I was just relieved to be out of pain.*

S Have you noticed anything else wrong recently?

P *No I don't think so. Like what?*

S Any changes with your bowels or any weight loss?

P *No.*

S How is your appetite then?

P *It seems normal to me.*

S Have you had any major diseases in the past or any operations?

P *I had my appendix out when I was eleven but I've always been as fit as a fiddle.*

S I'm just going to summarise what you have said to me. You are 35 years of age. Suddenly, whilst at work, you developed very severe pain in the outer part of your abdomen (points to site of pain), which seemed to shoot down into your groin. The pain lasted a few minutes at a time and was sharp. It made you want to roll around. The pain kept coming but eventually disappeared when you had an injection in accident and emergency. You now feel fine?

P　*Yes that's exactly how it happened.*

S　Thank you very much for your help Mr Jones. I am now going to speak to my consultant about your problem and we can arrange some investigations for you.

E　What do you think is this patient's diagnosis?

S　I think he has ureteric colic.

E　What factors in this patient's history have led you to make that diagnosis?

S　The patient's age and sex, the short history of severe colic radiating from the loin to the groin and the history of dehydration.

E　What complications may arise as a result of this condition?

S　The patient may develop urinary infection, obstruction or ureteric strictures.

The bell sounds for the end of the station.

Comment

Abdominal pain is such a common symptom that any examiner in any undergraduate medical examination will expect you to take a competent history. This student handles the situation well in many ways. Even within the constraint of a 5-minute session, the student demonstrates their communication skills with the use of many open questions and finds time to empathise with the patient's concerns.

Ureteric colic is a very common problem. Normally it is caused by the formation of small stones in the renal pelvis. Dehydration will encourage the formation of stones because the urine will become solute rich and solvent depleted. Most stones (60–70%) are composed of calcium oxalate. Stones of magnesium ammonium phosphate make up the about 15–20% and the rest are composed of calcium phosphate (5%), uric acid (5%) and, finally, cystine (1%). Overall, about 90% of stones are radio-opaque.

Learning points

- Abdominal history is EXTREMELY common in undergraduate exams.
- You must demonstrate absolute familiarity with the structure of abdominal history.

- As you are taking the history, try to think around the subject, particularly if the patient volunteers information. In the above scenario, the patient spends some time describing his potential state of dehydration and this history gives a strong hint of diagnosis.
- If time is a factor, then start with the most important points and finish with the standard questions that are least likely to influence the diagnosis. In this 5-minute scenario, the examiner will understand that if given time, you would have proceeded to a more thorough review of systems and anaesthetic pre-assessment.
- Colic is a common symptom. By carefully focusing on severity and length of colic waves, a working diagnosis can be easily reached (see Table 2.1).

Station extension

In a longer station, the examiner may ask you how to investigate this patient. The initial investigations seek to clarify the diagnosis. Because 90% of ureteric stones are visible on plain X-ray, a plain abdominal X-ray (colloquially known as a kidney-ureter-bladder or KUB X-ray) should be ordered together with a urine dipstick for blood. Secondary investigations should include an intravenous urogram and serum calcium to look for occult hyperparathyroidism.

Suggestions for further practice

Time is of the essence in this sort of short OSCE station. You should time yourself taking short histories like this. Moreover, take the opportunity to record yourself taking such a history if you can. It is amazing how listening to yourself will highlight unnecessary pauses and stumbles in your history taking.

Rectal bleeding

Level:	*/**
Setting:	60-year-old man sat in a chair
Time:	5 minutes

Rectal bleeding is an exceptionally common symptom. It is a common OSCE station because of the diagnostic thought processes that are required to differentiate between life-threatening (e.g. rectal carcinoma) and less serious (e.g. haemorrhoids) pathology. Moreover, general surgeons appear to have an obsession with the symptom and it is easy to find such a surgeon who will teach the subject with enthusiasm. The source of the bleeding can be from any part of the GI tract.

Task

E   You are a pre-registration house officer (foundation-year trainee) in a colorectal outpatient clinic. Please take a history from this gentleman who has noticed some blood when he opens his bowels.

Response

Once again, although the instructions are specific, you must attempt to use the established structure of a surgical history; starting with the name, age and occupation of the patient, and proceeding to presenting complaint and history of presenting complaint, etc. The patient may perceive rectal bleeding as embarrassing and you must presume that he is not used to talking about such intimate subjects. Thus, your communication skills are extremely important in such a scenario. Moreover, it is essential that, as the story becomes clear, your diagnostic thought processes focus on the key facts. This station illustrates to the examiner the ability of a highly competent student to compress a lengthy history into a very short time.

Rectal bleeding

Rectal bleeding typically presents in one of two ways:

- Small volume recurrent and chronic
- Single large volume and acute

Because the site of bleeding is close to the anal margin, the blood is usually seen as bright red. Bleeding from haemorrhoids or an anal fissure is invariably related to defecation. These are more commonly seen in younger patients. Pain tends to be the predominant feature of anal fissure, whereas bleeding and prolapse predominate in haemorrhoids. A combination of recurrent rectal bleeding in young patients aged less than 40 years in association with peri-anal symptoms (pain, prolapse, pruritus) nearly always has a benign cause.

Blood mixed in with the substance of the stool is associated with a greater risk of malignancy. This is, in many ways, obvious because a cause of bleeding higher than the anal canal does give the blood an opportunity to mix with forming faeces.

Patients with carcinoma and colitis often pass just blood and mucus alone, without accompanying faecal matter and this symptom almost always indicates significant disease in the rectum or left colon. Patients with these pathologies are also likely to have a change in bowel habit, with a looser stool and abdominal pain. Again age is a useful discriminator; patients under the age of 40 years are more likely to have colitis, whilst patients older than this are more likely to have malignant disease.

It is a common misconception that diverticular disease presents with recurrent bleeding. This is rarely the case. Occasionally, patients with diverticulitis can present with a brisk or sometimes catastrophic bleed, but this is rare. Bleeding from infectious causes is rare in the UK because the infectious organisms rarely cause ulceration of the mucosa.

In summary, patients with recurrent low-volume bleeding:

- age < 40 years + peri-anal symptoms = benign disease
- age > 40 years + change of bowel habit + blood mixed with stool = likelihood of malignancy.

For patients with benign disease:

- pain predominates = fissure
- prolapse and bleeding = haemorrhoids.

In patients who present with a large acute bleed, you should consider:

- angiodysplasia
- diverticular disease
- ischaemic colitis
- over-anticoagulation and other clotting abnormalities (but likely to be 'unmasking' another cause)
- rarely, carcinoma and inflammatory bowel disease.

As this sort of acute bleeding often originates from higher in the colon, the blood is more likely to be dark red and mixed with the stool. It can even resemble melaena[4], but does not have quite as unpleasant a smell, nor is it truly black. In over 90% of cases, the bleeding will settle spontaneously. After the bleeding has stopped, the colon should be investigated to exclude colitis, carcinoma or post-ischaemic stricture. Recurrent large-volume bleeding is rare. If the bleeding does not stop, intervention is required with colonoscopy or angiography. Both of these procedures can be diagnostic and therapeutic. Resection of the affected segment is required if these techniques are ineffective.

51

---

[4] Melaena is from the Greek melaina, which is the feminine form of melas=black and means "the passage of dark, pitchy and grumous stools stained with blood pigments or with altered blood"

GASTROINTESTINAL

Station extensions

You may be asked how you would investigate such a patient and then shown a photograph of the relevant investigation. Commonly this will be a proctoscopy, sigmoidoscopy or flexible colonoscopy showing a specific pathology. It is unlikely that you will be asked the specifics of surgical intervention, because this is frequently complex and rarely required.

Suggestions for further practice

Make sure that you have seen several proctoscopies, rigid sigmoidoscopies and flexible sigmoidoscopies. Revise the anatomy of the large bowel and be familiar with the normal appearance of the anus, rectum and colon. There are several commercially available videos of rectal/colonic investigations and most good medical libraries will have a selection.

Presenting a history of rectal bleeding

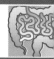

Level:	*/**
Setting:	Single examiner
Time:	5 minutes

Scenario

You have just taken a 5-minute history from a 70-year-old man with a 3-month history of rectal bleeding:

E Please present the patient's history to me

S Mr Smith is a 70-year-old retired joiner who sought advice from his GP about 2 weeks ago. Three months ago he noticed that his stool had a small streak of blood mixed in with it. At that time he had no other symptoms, but over the course of the last 3 months his bowels have become looser and he's noticed more and more blood. He is opening his bowels about three times a day at the moment. The stool is well formed, but there are streaks of blood every time. He has not noticed any blood separate from his stool and he does not complain of inadvertent soiling. There is no associated abdominal pain. He says that his stool does not have an unusual smell.

He says that over the last 6 weeks he has noticed his clothes becoming looser and his wife has commented that he has lost weight. About 3 weeks ago he noticed that after each bowel movement there was a sensation of tenesmus[5] and for the last 3 days he has noticed some air bubbles in his urine. He also complains of tiredness and lethargy over the last 6 weeks or so.

He had a cholecystectomy in 1990 and was investigated in 1980 for a duodenal ulcer but is otherwise fit and well. His grandfather died aged 71 with secondary cancer, which the patient thinks started in his bowel. He does not smoke and drinks small quantities of alcohol and lives with his wife who is fit and well. He has two children and six grandchildren. A review of other systems was unremarkable. Mr Smith is very concerned that he may have cancer.

Comment

This is a very competent presentation and illustrates a student with advanced cognitive and diagnostic thought. The student gives a detailed chronological and relevant history of the presenting complaint and by the time he reports weight loss the diagnosis is clear. As he is reasonably confident about the diagnosis,

---

[5] Teinesmos is from the Greek teinein, to strain, stretch

53

he has not reported symptoms which may be relevant to other causes of rectal bleeding such as pruritus or anal pain. In addition, he presents only the associated symptoms that are relevant to a diagnosis of suspected carcinoma. The final line in the presentation indicates to the examiner the student's concern for the patient's general well-being.

The examiner continues:

E   What do you think is Mr Smith's diagnosis?

S   I think it is likely that Mr Smith has a rectal or recto-sigmoid carcinoma.

E   How do you explain the bubbles in his urine?

S   I think that it is likely that this is pneumaturia from a recto-vesical fistula.

Comment

The examiner asks this question to assess the students understanding of the potential complications of a rectal cancer. This is a tough line of questioning for an average student, because it is a relatively rare condition. If the student stumbled at this point, it is likely that the examiner would understand and provide some helpful suggestions.

E   How can the diagnosis of rectal carcinoma be confirmed?

S   In the first instance, I would perform a thorough examination including a rectal examination.

E   What instruments might be used to aid the rectal examination?

S   Rigid sigmoidoscopy in the first instance.

E   How likely is it, do you think, that you would be able to see a rectal carcinoma using a rigid sigmoidoscope?

S   Very likely.

E   And a carcinoma was seen, what would be performed?

S   A small biopsy would be taken.

E   How do you explain Mr Smith's lethargy and malaise?

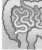

S Given the length of history and his current symptoms, I think Mr Smith is likely to be anaemic from chronic blood loss or from the anaemia associated with malignancy.

E What sort of anaemia is he likely to have?

S An iron-deficiency or hypochromic, microcytic anaemia.

The bell sounds for the end of the station.

This student has performed well. The responses to all the examiner's questions were succinct and accurate and it is difficult to see how this student would not have scored well.

Comment

Rectal carcinoma is a common condition. It is most often seen in Westernised countries. Because it is so prevalent and the mainstay of treatment is surgical, it is very frequently the subject of examination questions. It is a subject that you should know well. Regular follow-on questions include:

- Predisposing factors
- Gross and microscopic appearance
- Screening and family history
- Complications.

Learning point

Whenever you take a history, try presenting it to someone. The more experience you have at doing this, the more confident you will be during such an OSCE station. Perhaps the best people to present to are Senior House Officers or Speciality Registrars who themselves will be approaching higher exams. You will find that they will ask very pertinent, if hard, questions!

55

Suggestions for further practice

Although you will not be expected to perform a sigmoidoscopy, you will be expected to be familiar with the technique, its uses and limitations. We would strongly suggest that you attend a colorectal diagnostic clinic and a lower-GI endoscopy list prior to your OSCE.

History of a lump in the neck

Level:	**/***
Setting:	45-year-old female patient
Time:	5 minutes

Task

You are asked to take a history from a 45-year-old woman with a swelling in her neck. You are a house-officer (foundation-year-1 trainee) in a hospital outpatient clinic.

Comment

On the face of it, this station should be straightforward and you may wonder why we have rated it **/***. There are two reasons for this; firstly it is our experience that of all the common history stations, this is the most poorly completed in an OSCE setting; secondly, the neck represents an 'examiner's paradise' because of the amount of knowledge, understanding and reasoning that can be tested in one small area.

When you think about it, the neck can be a focus for assessing a candidate's knowledge of:

- *anatomy*: posterior and anterior triangle, cranial nerves, thyroid, thymus, lymph nodes, embryology, anatomical relationships and the effect of compression, etc.
- *physiology*: hypothalamo-pituitary-thyroid axis, functions, function and effects of thyroid hormones, parathyroid hormones, swallowing, laryngeal function, etc.
- *pathology*: thyroid and parathyroid disease, lymphatic disease, oesophageal abnormalities, cranial nerve abnormalities, carotid disease, etc.
- *systemic disease*: any disease that causes swelling of the cervical lymph nodes, generalised arteriopathy, etc.

Further consideration will tell you that this list is by no means exhaustive! Having said this, thyroid lumps and cervical lymph nodes appear most commonly in clinical examinations because of their relatively high incidence.

Narrow down your options

In a 5-minute station, it is ESSENTIAL that you narrow down your field of enquiry as early as you can during your history to avoid being taken away from the underlying diagnosis. Consider the flow chart (Figure 6). Asking the three

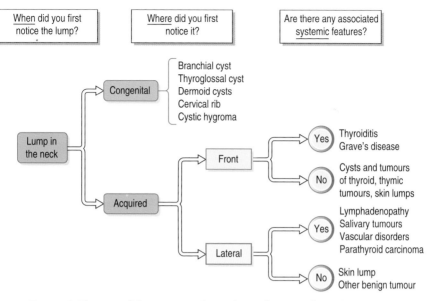

Figure 6 Three useful questions when taking a history of a neck swelling

questions: 'When did you first notice it?', 'Where in your neck is it?' and 'Is there anything else you have noticed about yourself', should help in rapidly narrowing down the potential diagnoses that you can then pursue in much greater depth.

Other important points in the history

The duration of symptoms is important in reaching a diagnosis; inflammatory conditions tend to develop and settle quite rapidly. Cervical lymphadenitis often is associated with recent upper-respiratory-tract infection. In contrast, congenital masses such as branchial or thyroglossal cysts are often present for an extended duration, sometimes since birth. Any malignant causes, such as metastatic carcinoma or primary lymphoma, tend to have a history of progressive unremitting growth. If it becomes clear early on in the history that the mass is likely to represent cervical lymphadenopathy, then associated symptoms need to be sought, so a review of systems will be helpful. For example, a history of weight loss over several months is much more likely to be associated with malignancy than an acute infection. Unfortunately, there are many causes of cervical lymphadenopathy (see Table 3.2) and, therefore, a thorough review of systems is necessary. Eighty per cent of malignant nodes in the neck are secondary to cancers in the upper aerodigestive system, and a history of smoking and alcohol usage should raise suspicion.

Further practice

Because neck lumps are so difficult, it is wise to spend considerable time thinking about how you might answer such a question. Try to construct a table

57

like the one in history 6, to see if you can pick out the differences in historical features that you would be likely to observe with the common causes of neck lump. Many large hospitals now have diagnostic 'one-stop' clinics for neck lumps, which are extremely useful for practising history taking and examination of patients.

Table 3.2 Causes of an enlarged cervical lymph node

Type	Specific cause	Rare (R) or common (C)
Bacterial	Infections of scalp or face (particularly β haemolytic *Strep.* and *Staph. aureus*)	C
	Actinomycosis	R
	Tuberculosis	C/R[6]
Viral	Upper respiratory tract infection	C
	Epstein–Barr infection	R
	HIV infection	R
	Herpes simplex	R
	Cytomegalovirus	R
Parasitic	*Toxoplasma gondii*	R
Fungal	*Coccioidomycosis*	R
Malignant	Primary lymphoma	C
	Secondary malignancy (particularly head and neck/bronchus)	C

[6] Highly dependent on geographical location

Upper GI bleeding

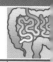

Level:	*/**
Setting:	50-year-old male patient
Time:	5 minutes

Task

You are a house officer (foundation-year-1 trainee) admitting a patient who has been vomiting blood. Please take a history.

Response

The presentation of upper-GI bleeding ranges from very minor to life-threatening haemorrhage. The station tests your ability to estimate the likely cause of the bleeding, the amount of blood lost and to diagnose shock.

Blood is a very good emetic and purgative. Most of the blood lost into the gut is passed out rapidly either in the vomit or faeces. Therefore, volume and frequency provide a good estimate of blood loss.

Specific aspects of history

- **Is it pure blood?** Ask if it was just blood, mixed with vomit, altered in colour (does it look like coffee grounds) or even just flecks.
- **How much?** Ask the patient to judge volumes in accordance with standard recognisable quantities such as a thimble, eggcup, cup, mug or jug. Haematemesis and melaena is usually associated with more blood loss than either alone. About 100–200 ml of blood in the upper GI tract is required to produce melaena. This may continue for several days after severe haemorrhage and does not necessarily indicate continued bleeding. Patients with chronic blood loss may present occasionally with symptoms and signs of anaemia (e.g. weakness, easy fatigability, pallor, chest pain, dizziness). In patients with cirrhosis, GI bleeding may precipitate hepatic encephalopathy (mental status changes secondary to liver failure).
- **What are the systemic effects?** Has the patient felt light headed, lost consciousness or collapsed? When present, all imply greater blood loss.
- **Estimate quantity.** Estimate which category your patient comes into: small (< 2 units blood), moderate (2–3 units) or large (> 3 units) haemorrhage so that when you present the history you can judge if the patient requires emergency or urgent treatment or alternatively just requires routine investigation.

GASTROINTESTINAL

Cause of Haematemesis

- **Peptic ulceration**. Ninety per cent of upper GI bleeds are as a result of peptic ulceration. Remember to ask about dyspepsia, antacid use, periodicity, non-steroidal anti-inflammatory drug and steroid use, previous history of peptic ulcer disease and family history. Don't worry about trying to differentiate gastric and duodenal ulcer, for example, by asking about relationship of the dyspepsia to food; this is not helpful.
- **Mallory–Weiss tear**. If patient vomits persistently before the bleeding starts, this is more likely.
- **Oesophageal varices**. Ask about alcohol consumption and history of liver disease.
- **Upper GI malignancy**. Ask about history of dysphagia and weight loss. Gastric carcinoma sometimes presents with haematemesis.
- **Bleeding diathesis**. Remember to ask about anticoagulant and anti-platelet therapy and history of bleeding disorders.

Altered bowel habit

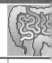

Level:	*/**
Setting:	Take a history from a standardised patient
Time:	5 minutes

Task

You are a final-year medical student attending a GP surgery. This patient has a change in bowel habit; you have to explore it as thoroughly as possible in 5 minutes.

S Good afternoon, my name is John Smith and I am a medical student. I have been asked by your doctor to ask you some questions. Is this OK?

P *Yes of course.*

S Can I start by asking your name and age?

P *John Davidson and I'm 61.*

S Thank you Mr Davidson. Now can you tell me about the problem that has brought you here today?

P *Yes I've been getting diarrhoea.*

Comment

The terms diarrhoea and constipation mean different things to different people. It is very important to clarify **exactly** what the patient means by these terms.

S Could you tell me more about your diarrhoea?

61

Comment

This is a good question, as well as being 'open' it is also non-patronising. It is so easy to irritate the patient by using phrases like "what do you mean by diarrhoea?" or even worse "diarrhoea means something completely different to doctors than it means to you".

P *I'm going to the toilet more often than I used to do.*

Comment

You must now establish if the bowel habit has **genuinely** changed and the **details** of the change.

S How often are you opening your bowels at the moment?

P *Oh about five times a day.*

S And what is normal for you?

P *For years I only opened my bowels once every other day.*

S When do you open your bowels?

P *Through the day normally, but over the last few weeks I have occasionally had to get up in the middle of the night.*

Comment

Nocturnal defecation is more likely to be associated with organic pathology.

S When you pass a stool, what is it like?

P *It used to be firm and brown but now it seems to be yellow, a bit slimy and quite watery at times.*

Comment

You must work within the structure of the medical history, use good communication skills; listen to the patient's own story and apply knowledge to focus and enquire about key factual details. The station illustrates how a competent student can elicit the key elements of the history in a short period of time.

S When did your bowels start to misbehave?

P *I first noticed a problem about three months ago.*

S And how have things changed since then?

P *Well my bowels are open more frequently now and sometimes I get some pain.*

Comment

Chronology is an essential part of surgical history taking. Very long and very short histories of change in bowel habit are less likely to be significant. Understanding the chronology greatly aids understanding the clinical problem and potential causes for the symptoms. Try asking, 'when did you notice a change in your bowel habit?' If the answer is not clear, suggest time limits, 'were your bowels normal 6 months ago/6 weeks ago' etc.? Obtain information on the following:

- Time course of the illness
- Any apparent precipitant
- Background factors
- Known previous or existing gastrointestinal disease
- Previous gastrointestinal history
- Family history of gastrointestinal disease
- Drug and alcohol disease.

Information about related symptoms

Change in bowel habit more often relates to pathology in the lower GI tract than the upper GI tract. Start with symptoms related to the lower bowel first and finish with a review of the upper GI tract.

Establish the presence of:

- blood and mucus. Is the blood mixed with the stool (inflammatory bowel disease, colonic/rectal tumours)?

- abdominal pain and relationship of the pain to the bowel habit. For example does the passage of stool alleviate or exacerbate the pain? Does eating exacerbate the pain (typical of partial small bowel obstruction, e.g. Crohn's)?
- abdominal distension (large bowel obstruction/ascites)
- tenesmus (rectal tumours)
- incontinence (faecal impaction/rectal masses).

Suggestions for further practice

Obtaining a good history of change of bowel habit can be a difficult skill to master. Given that enquiry about bowel habit is part of a standard review of systems, you should take this opportunity in getting used to defining 'normal' bowel habit (you will be amazed at how variable 'normal' is in the general population). Talking about bowel habit can be embarrassing for both student and patient. If enquiry about bowel habit becomes routine to you, the embarrassment will be relieved for both you and the patient. This is because you will learn to use language and phraseology which the patient can understand. It is not unusual for the patient to believe that you have gone mad when you ask them about their last 'stool'!

Core skill   **History of altered bowel habit**

You should be able to answer the following questions in presenting the history:

Has the bowel habit really changed?

How has it changed?

What is the chronology (time problems started and change over time)?

What are the related symptoms?

   blood and mucus

   abdominal pain

   tenesmus

   incontinence

   weight loss

   anorexia

What background factors may be related?

   pre-existing GI disease

   family history of GI disease

   drug and alcohol usage

   usual diet

Painless jaundice

Level:	**
Setting:	Take a history from a standardised patient
Time:	10 minutes

Task

E You are a student on a surgical ward. This is Mr Jones. I would like you to take a history from him. After a while I will stop you and ask you some questions.

Comment

This type of station is regularly used in some schools. The idea is that you will extract a brief history and the examiner will use the second half of the station to link your history-taking skills to your knowledge of a particular group of symptoms.

S Hello Mr Jones. I'm very pleased to meet you. My name is Jim, I'm a final-year medical student and I would like to ask you some questions. Is that OK?

P *Fire away!*

S How old are you?

P *70 last June.*

S Could you first tell me what seems to be the problem that has brought you into hospital?

P *Yes, it's fascinating. I was having Christmas dinner 6 weeks ago with my kids and grandchildren and my 7-year-old granddaughter Livvy said that I was a funny colour. I asked her what she meant and she said I looked yellow. Sure enough my son agreed with her and within a couple of days I was bright yellow. I mean I felt well enough.*

S Did you notice anything else about yourself?

P *Well my wife said that she thought I had lost a bit of weight but apart from the normal aches and pains of old age I felt fine.*

S When you say 'normal aches and pains' what did you mean?

P *Well I always have pains in my knees and a bit of back pain. In fact my back has been quite troublesome for a few months now but it's not affecting me particularly.*

Comment

This last bit of dialogue will impress an examiner because the student has picked up on a clue, which the patient sees as normal, but may be relevant to the diagnosis.

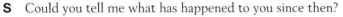

S Could you tell me what has happened to you since then?

P *I went to see my GP and he did some blood tests. About 3 days later I had a phone call from the local hospital asking me to come in urgently because I was jaundiced. I was still yellow and losing weight.*

S And then what happened?

P *I came into hospital and they did some tests on me and got rid of my jaundice.*

S Do you know how they got rid of it?

P *Yes they put me to sleep and put a telescope down my mouth.*

E OK I'll stop you there I am going to ask you some questions. How would you summarise Mr Jones' problems?

S Mr Jones is a 70-year-old man who developed painless jaundice about 6 weeks ago. The jaundice was associated with some weight loss and perhaps some back pain. He was subsequently admitted to hospital for investigation.

E What are the common causes of painless jaundice? You can speak openly because Mr Jones is a simulated patient.

S The commonest causes are carcinoma of the head of the pancreas, viral hepatitis, hepatic metastases and alcoholic cirrhosis. Oh and gallstones in the common bile duct can be painless too. There are several rarer causes.

Table 3.3 Causes of painless jaundice

Common	Viral hepatitis
	Carcinoma of the head of the pancreas
	Hepatic metastases
	Alcoholic cirrhosis
	Gallstones in common bile duct
Less common	Alcoholic hepatitis
	Primary biliary cirrhosis
	Drugs (e.g. chlorpromazine)
	Haemolytic anaemia
	Venous congestion from heart failure
	Cholangitis and pancreatitis
Rare	Carcinoma of the bile duct
	Inherited hyperbilirubinaemia
	Cholestasis of pregnancy

GASTROINTESTINAL

E Which do you think is most likely in Mr Jones and why?

S Given Mr Jones' age, weight loss, back pain and his story since he came into hospital, I would think the most likely diagnosis is carcinoma of the head of the pancreas.

E Why is he not jaundiced now?

S From his description, he sounds like he has had an ERCP and a stent inserted.

E What is an ERCP?

S An ERCP is an endoscopic retrograde cholangio-pancreaticogram.

E And what function does it serve?

S It uses a special side-viewing endoscope, which can look directly into the duodenum. Contrast medium can be injected into the bile ducts to look for abnormalities.

E Is an ERCP just an investigation then?

S It can also be used to treat a patient. For instance, a stent can be inserted down the endoscope to bypass an obstruction.

E Well done. You are correct; it appears as though Mr Jones does have carcinoma of the head of the pancreas. Why does this tumour cause biliary obstruction?

S The head of the pancreas sits in the natural curve of the duodenum. The pancreatic duct merges with the common bile duct, next to the head of the pancreas, just before these tubes open into the second part of the duodenum at the ampulla of Vater[7]. Any growth at this site will tend to obstruct the common bile duct.

E What further tests would you like to perform on Mr Jones?

S I would like to investigate the tumour itself.

E How would you do this?

66

---

[7] Abraham Vater (1684–1751) Professor of Anatomy and Botany, University of Wittenberg

S   Initially I would arrange an abdominal ultrasound, but CT or MRI scans would probably give a more detailed assessment of the pancreas and biliary system.

E   Mr Jones had a CT scan last Tuesday. This is the report.

> **Box 3.3 X-RAY Department**
> **University Hospital of St Elsewhere**
>
> CT abdomen
>
> In the head of the pancreas is a 2 cm well-circumscribed mass. It has irregular margins and lies close to the pancreatic and common bile ducts. There are no obvious signs of metastases. Appearance is consistent with a carcinoma.

E   What do you think should be done now?

S   Because the tumour is well circumscribed and there are no obvious signs of metastases, Mr Jones may benefit from resection of the tumour.

Comment

This student has answered this station very well. In fact most examiners would not be expecting the quality of responses that this candidate gave to the supplemental questions. The student is succinct and does not wander off from the point of the station at any time. The station also illustrates the importance of 'reading around' a subject; a good answer requires **integration** of clinical skills with clinical and basic science knowledge.

Station extensions

The possibilities for extending this station are wide-ranging but consider:

- liver function tests in a patient with obstructive jaundice
- issues around palliative care of somebody with non-resectable abdominal cancer
- radiological image picture of the common bile duct.

Suggestions for further practice

As well as attending endoscopy sessions where patients are investigated for jaundice, this station illustrates how important it is to understand what you are seeing when you are watching a complex skill like ERCP. It is a golden rule when learning surgery (like many other clinical subjects) that, as soon as you can after seeing a procedure, you reinforce what you have seen with the relevant knowledge to enable you to **understand** it. When you are preparing for an OSCE, it is insufficient to simply learn a skill without such understanding.

Painful leg (vascular)

Level:	**
Setting:	Take a history from a standardised patient
Time:	10 minutes

Task

You are a final-year medical student who has been asked to take a history from this patient who is complaining of pain in his legs when he walks.

Comment

If the average medical student is examined in five/six OSCEs during his/her clinical years, it is virtually certain that one of the stations will include taking a history from a patient with lower-limb vascular insufficiency. The reasons for this are:

- it is a very common condition
- it is chronic
- many of the patients are elderly and willing to participate in student examinations.

We will discuss in depth the examination of such a patient later, but in this section we will briefly discuss the important diagnostic aspects of the history. Once again, vascular diagnosis depends quite heavily on a basic understanding of the anatomy of the peripheral vascular system. The principal cause of vascular injury in Western Society is arterial narrowing and occlusion due to atherosclerosis. Symptoms depend on the site of narrowing, thus anatomical knowledge is important.

The following points are particularly important in a vascular history:

1. Patient age and sex

The prevalence of peripheral arterial disease of the legs in men (assessed by non-invasive tests) is about 3% in people younger than 60 years, but rises to greater than 20% in people older than 75 years[8].

2. Pain

The primary task of a doctor assessing arterial insufficiency is to determine if the patient has reached a stage that is critical to the survival of the limb. This so-called critical ischaemia represents a vascular surgical urgency and urgent

---

[8] Fowkes FG, Housley E, Cawood EH et al. Edinburgh Artery Study: prevalence of asymptomatic and symptomatic peripheral arterial disease in the general population. Int J Epidemiol 1991;20:384–92

investigation and management is necessary. The pain of critical ischaemia is characteristically severe, constant and occurs at rest.

Once the possibility of critical ischaemia has been eliminated (a scenario unlikely to be met in an OSCE exam, because of the need for urgent treatment), then the history of pain is used to determine the degree of vascular insufficiency in combination with the restrictions that the disease is having on the patient's quality of life.

Classically, intermittent claudication develops following a period of exercise (normally walking) and is relieved, rapidly, by rest. This is followed by a period where the patient can walk the same distance before getting pain again.

The site of pain will help determine the site of the lesion.

- **Bilateral, entire leg:** aorta
- **Buttock and thigh:** external and internal iliac
- **Thigh and calf:** external iliac/common femoral.
- **Calf pain:** superficial femoral/popliteal.

The pain is characteristically cramping and varies from an ache to severe, disabling pain. The claudication distance (distance walked on a flat surface before the onset of pain) should be estimated.

Box 3.4 Critical ischaemia definition[9]

Persistently recurring ischaemic rest pain requiring regular adequate analgesia for more than 2 weeks, or ulceration or gangrene of the foot or toes, with an ankle pressure of < 50 mmHg or toe pressure of < 30 mmHg.

[9] European Working Group on Critical Leg Ischaemia 1991

69

3. Associated symptoms

Ask about changes in skin, ulcers or sores in the lower limb. Have they been seeing a chiropodist regularly? Is there paraesthesia or any signs of Raynaud's phenomenon? In males, ask about their sexual history (erections).

4. Review of systems

Vascular surgeons consider PVD to be symptomatic of whole-body arteriopathy; PVD is an independent risk factor for ischaemic heart disease, strokes and hypertension. Intermittent claudication carries a 3–4–fold increase in mortality from myocardial infarction or strokes. Ask about each of these in detail. Specifically ask about:

- diabetes mellitus
- hypertension
- hyperlipidaemia
- family history.

CARDIOVASCULAR

5. Smoking history

About 30% of the UK population are currently heavy smokers. In patients with intermittent claudication, > 95% are, or have been, heavy smokers (> 20 cigarettes per day for > 15 years = 15 pack years).

6. Effect on quality of life

In one sense, this is the most important information you can gain. This is mainly because most vascular surgeons now will not consider surgery on patients with claudication that has a minimal or moderate effect on quality of life. This is because the patients are subjected to long, complicated surgical procedures with high failure rates, which can leave them symptomatically worse. You want to know if the patient has regular employment and if his symptoms affect this. You must also enquire about normal activities of daily living.

E   What investigations would you perform on someone with a recent onset of claudication? His claudication distance is 200 yards.

Comment

Although this is an obvious follow-up question, the answer is controversial. Initially all patients should have the following baseline tests:

- Plasma glucose
- Full blood count for anaemia or polycythaemia (may exacerbate symptoms)
- Random cholesterol
- ESR to eliminate an inflammatory vasculitis
- ECG and chest radiograph to look for other signs of vascular disease
- Doppler estimation of ankle/brachial pressure index (ABPI). An ABPI of between 0.5 and 0.8 suggests significant arterial occlusion
- Peripheral lower limb arteriography. Although this remains the definitive investigation for PVD, it is not without risks. Today most surgeons reserve arteriography for those patients in whom they would consider interventional radiological or surgical treatment.

E   How would you manage someone with intermittent claudication?

Comment

As in all surgical situations management can be divided into conservative, medical and surgical.

Amputation

Amputation is performed for diseased limbs when attempts at salvage and reconstruction may be lengthy, emotionally and financially costly, and have a less-than-satisfactory result. Indications for limb removal include:

Table 3.4 Management of lower limb ischaemia

Conservative	Smoking cessation
	Weight loss
	Careful foot care/chiropody
	Take regular controlled aerobic exercise
Drugs	Lipid-lowering therapy
	Optimise treatment of diabetes and cardiac function
	Anti-platelet therapy
Surgical	Balloon angioplasty
	Reconstructive surgery
	Amputation

- severe peripheral vascular disease
- trauma
- infection
- congenital abnormalities.

The leading indication for limb amputation in the UK and most of the Western world is peripheral vascular disease. Patients with diabetes mellitus account for nearly 50% of the population with PVD.

Indications for lower-limb amputation in patients with PVD are:

- uncontrollable soft tissue or bone infection
- non-reconstructable disease with persistent tissue loss
- unrelenting rest pain due to muscle ischaemia.

There are numerous forms of lower-limb amputation, but the ones you are likely to see are below and above knee and trans-metatarsal. The optimum site of amputation is determined by **two** basic surgical principles:

- make a stump that will heal
- make the stump as distal as possible to maintain maximum function.

Station extensions

Patients with PVD are frequently the subjects of longer stations in OSCEs.

You may be:

- shown a lower-limb arteriogram and asked to comment on the findings
- asked to describe the social impact on patients with PVD/lower-limb amputation
- asked to discuss smoking cessation with the patient.

CARDIOVASCULAR

Suggestions for further practice

- Visit a diabetic or vascular clinic and take detailed histories from patients with PVD
- Explore with PVD patients the effect of their disease on the quality of life
- Arrange to observe an arteriogram being performed.

Core skill	History of pain

1. Site: ask the patient to point
2. Radiation: does the pain seem to move
3. Character: sharp, dull, 'like toothache', stabbing, crushing
4. Severity: "on a scale of 1 to 10 with 1 being a slight niggle and 10 being the worst pain you could imagine"
5. Duration: how long has the pain been present? Constant or variable?
6. Frequency: does the pain appear regularly – is it 'phasic'?
7. Aggravating factors: movement, staying still, walking, sitting, climbing stairs
8. Relieving factors: drugs, rest, exercise
9. Associated features: stiffness, swelling, locking, altered sensation

Painful limb (orthopaedic)

Level:	*
Setting:	70-year-old male patient lying on an examination couch
Time:	10 minutes

Task

You are asked to take a history from an elderly man who is complaining of pain in his leg and a limp. He is lying on a couch and is holding a walking stick.

S Hello Sir (shakes hands). My name is Joan Smith and I am a final-year medical student. May I ask you some questions?

P *Yes of course, what would you like to know?*

S May I ask your name and how old you are?

P *Peter Jones and I'm seventy next month.*

S Would you describe the problem that has been troubling you?

P *There are several things really.*

S OK. Start from the beginning and please take your time.

Comment

The informality and openness of this introduction informs the examiner that the student is comfortable in this environment. The concern is that, in an OSCE, asking the patient to start from the beginning may be hazardous because some patients may take this as a cue to tell you about things that are irrelevant to their current condition. However, an experienced and capable clinician will recognise the digression quickly and gently ease the patient back on track.

P *About 3 years ago I started to get a pain sort of round my right knee. (Patient uses the palm of his hand to rub his knee and lower thigh.)*

Comment

The use of the hand to describe pain can be a valuable source of information. Use of the palm here tends to suggest that the pain is not localised and one may guess that if the patient was asked to point to the pain with one finger he would struggle to do so.

P *Over the last few years it seems to have got worse and worse, and in recent weeks the pain seems to have moved up my leg and I can now feel it here. (Patient points to groin on right). I really struggle to walk and my doctor sent me here for some X-rays.*

S What is the pain like?

73

LOCOMOTOR

P   *It's difficult to describe really. It nags at me all the time like a toothache. It gets me down.*

Comment

The patient has volunteered information about the psychological sequelae of the pain and this should not be ignored. The tendency in the heat of the OSCE is to ignore such cues and carry on with your history structure. Try to acknowledge the way the patient feels.

S   It must be very difficult for you.

P   *Oh it's terrible at times. It's on my mind all the time, gnawing away at me and it seems to be getting worse and worse.*

S   You said it was terrible at times. What did you mean by that?

P   *It's particularly bad just before I go to bed and it's uncomfortable to walk any great distance. It's stopping me doing all sorts of things I used to be able to do.*

S   What sorts of things would they be?

P   *I've started to have to walk with a stick if I'm going outside. I can't tie my own shoelaces and I'm starting to find dressing a struggle.*

S   How far can you walk at the moment?

P   *I can normally get about half a mile on the flat, but it is very difficult to get up the stairs.*

S   Why is tying your shoelaces so difficult? Is it because of the pain?

P   *Not really. It's more like I just can't. I'm just so stiff.*

S   Does anything seem to make the pain better?

P   *It is easier when I get up in the morning and after I've had a rest. My GP gave me some of these (holding packet of ibuprofen) and they work for an hour or so and then the pain comes back.*

Comment

The student in this scenario appears to have taken a thorough history of the presenting complaint. Given that this is a 10-minute station, you should now be thinking about what else is important to find out before you present your history at the next station! Although this patient's presentation is slightly atypical (most patients with osteoarthritis of the hip present with pain in the groin and down the front of the thigh) the remaining presenting complaint is highly suggestive of:

- a non-inflammatory condition (worse at night and exercise)
- a focal problem in the hip not the knee (pain is localised around one joint and no other joints appear to be causing problems).

As a rule of thumb OSCE stations involving osteoarthritis are more likely to have an orthopaedic surgical focus, particularly OA of the hip and knee, whilst inflammatory arthritides are more likely to have a rheumatological focus.

Most patients who are accessible to take part in an examination with OA are waiting for, or have had, joint replacement. A 'test wise' student who is taking a history like the one above, will be prepared for a surgical rather than a medical discussion, either at the end of the station or at the next station, where she will be asked to present the history she has just taken. With this in mind, during the remaining time, the student should concentrate on:

- the patient's fitness for a general anaesthetic
- the specific degree of functional limitation
- the social and psychological impact of the disorder
- problems that may impede recovery from surgery.

Fitness for anaesthesia

As discussed in Chapter 1, assessment of fitness for anaesthesia and surgery is a basic competence required for all surgical foundation trainees. Recent studies of elective hip replacement reveal a mortality of about 1:700, with most of these patients dying within 30 days.

Risk factors for mortality were increased age, being male, and a history of cardio-respiratory disease. The low mortality compares very favourably to the rates that were reported when hip replacement first became popular using the Charnley[11] hip prosthesis in 1962. Much of this improved mortality has come from improved patient selection facilitated by more accurate and predictive pre-operative assessment. Your history should cover the following areas:

- **Patients mental state and mobility** will influence the type of anaesthetic used. Regional anaesthesia may be inappropriate for a confused patient or a patient who is unable to lie flat.
- **A review of organ systems** with particular reference to cardiovascular and respiratory problems. Much of the role of an anaesthetist administering an anaesthetic involves the support of the patient's cardiac and respiratory systems. In fit and healthy patients, both of these systems have considerable reserve and can withstand considerable artificial stresses put upon them by general anaesthesia. Therefore, it is important to gather as much information about the patient's cardiac and respiratory health prior to such anaesthesia. A history of cough, angina, myocardial infarction and smoking should be carefully ascertained. Patients who cannot move well because of joint problems may have very limited cardiovascular reserve, but, because they cannot exert themselves, these may be hidden. Such patients may require specialised investigations, such as lung function testing or echocardiography before surgery.
- **Drug history** - warfarin, aspirin and non-steroidal anti-inflammatory drugs (NSAIDs) have side-effects, such as upper gastrointestinal bleeding, renal toxicity and platelet dysfunction and may prevent the anaesthetist

75

---

[11] Sir John Charnley (1911–1982) Surgeon from Wrightington, Manchester, UK

LOCOMOTOR

from performing an epidural. Many elderly patients are on cardiovascular treatment, particularly beta-blockers and ACE-inhibitors, and these may adversely affect cardiovascular stability during anaesthesia.

- **Diabetes**: patients with impaired glucose tolerance pose a particular problem for the anaesthetist. Surgery produces a catabolic state and patients have to starve for a period of time prior to surgery to prevent aspiration of stomach contents. Moreover, the blood sugar of many patients with diabetes is controlled using drugs such as glicazide or long-acting insulin. Thus, diabetic patients have a significant susceptibility for the development of prolonged and life-threatening hypoglycaemia. Knowledge about the management of diabetes is necessary when oral intake is going to be restricted.
- **Allergies:**   antibiotics, anaesthetics, iodine, etc.
- **Past surgical history:**   any difficulties in spinal/epidural insertion, airway management, and other problems encountered.

Anaesthetists regularly use a number of grading systems in assessing anaesthetic risk. You should be familiar with the ASA system (see Table 3.5), which is the most commonly used. It is worth noting that ASA grade IV and V patients are rarely encountered in OSCEs!

Degree of functional, social and psychological limitation

The decision to surgically treat patients with degenerative joint disease relies very heavily on the functional impairment experienced by the patient and their quality of life. The specific indication for total hip replacement is severe pain and stiffness from arthritis in the hip, that limits an individual's ability to do the things they want to do. The decision to treat relies heavily on the patient's pre-existing quality of life and this has to be balanced with the risks of surgery and the improvement in quality of life that surgery is likely to bring. Quality of life is notoriously difficult to assess and you should focus your questioning on:

- how the patient feels about his/her disability
- the precise nature of his/her functional disability linked to his/her activities of daily living

Table 3.5 ASA[12] physical status classification

ASA I	Healthy patient
ASA II	Mild systemic disease with no functional limitation – for example, controlled hypertension
ASA III	Severe systemic disease with definite functional limitation – for example, chronic obstructive pulmonary disease
ASA IV	Severe systemic disease that is a constant threat to life – for example, unstable angina
ASA V	Moribund patient who is not expected to survive for 24 hours with or without surgery

[12] ASA = American Society of Anesthesiologists

- if the patient is depressed, anxious or filled with feelings of helplessness because of his/her incapacity
- if the disease has restricted employment
- whether the patient has trouble participating in everyday personal and family pleasures and responsibilities.

In addition you should be aware of contraindications for joint replacement surgery. This surgery is usually not recommended for:

- very young patients. This is because modern joint prostheses have a limited lifespan. 'Re-do' joint surgery is much more complicated than an initial replacement and has higher complication rates and surgical mortality
- patients with concurrent hip infection
- patients with a paralysed quadriceps muscles
- neurological disorders affecting the hip
- patients with severely limiting psychiatric disorders
- serious physical disease (terminal disease, such as metastatic cancer)
- extreme obesity (severe obesity BMI between 35 and 40, morbid obesity BMI>40).

How will the patient cope with recovery from surgery?

A careful assessment of the patient's living circumstances should be ascertained. Patients who live alone or who have no access to appropriate transport will need intervention from support agencies before discharge and during home-based rehabilitation.

General principles of orthopaedic history

As in almost all clinical scenarios, a thorough and comprehensive orthopaedic history is fundamental to accurate diagnosis. Perhaps not surprisingly, many students tend to neglect the orthopaedic history in the mistaken belief that a plain X-ray is THE essential diagnostic tool. In consequence, orthopaedic history, and to a lesser extent examination OSCE stations are frequently badly handled. It is true that orthopaedics, more than any other subject, utilises X-rays in the diagnostic process, but this is simply because bones are visible on X-rays and there are a lot of bones. They remain, however, only a type of diagnostic investigation and it would be foolhardy to base your orthopaedic revision entirely on X-rays. Orthopaedics is a complex subject that is also concerned with soft tissues such as tendons, ligaments and joints, which are not visible on a plain radiograph. The vast majority of elective orthopaedic operations are performed to correct abnormalities with these tissues rather than the bones.

Orthopaedic patients are very common subjects in OSCEs because many of the conditions are long-standing and very common. To complicate matters further, most joint problems occur in an elderly population; thus, the incidence of coexisting disease in these patients is high. Often these coexisting medical problems will influence orthopaedic management (e.g. an elderly patient with a very recent myocardial infarction is unlikely to undergo elective hip replacement quickly).

General rules for history taking

History taking in orthopaedics should differ little in its structure from that of any other subspecialty. However there are some areas of the standard history that are particularly relevant to orthopaedics.

- **Pain:** pain is the principal symptom of orthopaedic complaints. Like all pain it should be assessed in a standard fashion. In orthopaedic patients, pain is frequently referred. For example, hip pain may not be felt in the hip, but more often in the groin or the knee.
- **Stiffness:** stiffness can be defined as limited movement without associated pain, though pain frequently accompanies it. In patients with chronic lumbar disc prolapse, stiffness without pain may manifest itself as a difficulty in tying shoelaces after getting out of bed. Whilst in patients with ankylosing spondylitis, a similar stiffness may be felt at all times. Stiffness may show diurnal variation and inflammatory conditions more often present with stiffness after prolonged rest, such as immediately after waking (i.e. in the morning). This stiffness frequently reduces after exercising the affected joint.
- **Locking** is a sudden stiffness, which occurs whilst attempting to complete a specific movement. This is normally due to a loose body within the joint itself. Most commonly it occurs in the knee and this is often due to separation of articular cartilage from the joint surface or fragments of ruptured menisci.
- **Swelling:** a complaint of swelling should be treated like any other focal symptom. Your questions should be similar to those you would ask if the patient is in pain, i.e. site, severity, preceding factors (trauma) speed of onset, aggravating and relieving factors. The pattern of joint swelling can often aid diagnosis, In Reiters syndrome for example, the swelling tends to be asymmetrical, fleeting and involve the large joints of the limbs.
- **Deformity:** historically many orthopaedic deformities were so common due to poor nutrition, infection and birth trauma that many of them have colloquial names. Examples include club foot, hammer toe, knock knees, flat feet, humpback, bow legs, lobster claw and barrel chest. It is sensible and polite to describe these deformities in medical terms. Perhaps the most important clinical feature of deformity is progression. A progressive deformity indicates an active, potentially reversible, disease process.
- **Altered sensation:** paraesthesia (tingling, pins and needles)[10] is a common sensation that most of us experience from time to time normally after sitting or lying in the same position for a prolonged period. This sort of paraesthesia normally quickly resolves. Paraesthesia is normally caused by an alteration in neurological function of a nerve by direct pressure or by ischaemia. Direct pressure may be a result of encroachment or pressure from a neighbouring

---

[10] Para Greek = beside, aesthesia Greek = sensation

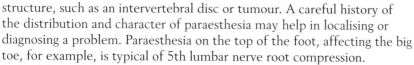

structure, such as an intervertebral disc or tumour. A careful history of the distribution and character of paraesthesia may help in localising or diagnosing a problem. Paraesthesia on the top of the foot, affecting the big toe, for example, is typical of 5th lumbar nerve root compression.

- **Loss of function:** loss of function can be absolute or relative. Absolute loss of function implies tissue damage that has resulted in a complete inability to perform a movement. A patient who has a traumatic rupture of the extensor tendons of the fingers CANNOT extend the fingers under any circumstances even if there is no accompanying pain. Relative loss of function depends on patient perception and normal activity. For example, a long-distance runner may complain of loss of function if he has sustained a bruise to the Achilles tendon, whilst a similar injury would probably not affect the daily functioning of a typical medical student!

In addition to these special considerations for the orthopaedic patient, fitness for anaesthesia, past medical and surgical history, social circumstances and quality of life are as important in patients with orthopaedic problems as in any other illness.

Back pain

Level:	**/***
Setting:	40-year-old male patient in a bed
Time:	10 minutes

Any GP will tell you that back pain is common and is often well represented amongst those whom the GP would classify as 'heart sink' patients. Many of the difficulties experienced by clinicians in the management of back pain arise because of the difficulty in arriving at a specific and accurate diagnosis. Back pain is particularly difficult because:

- different underlying pathologies can present with very similar symptoms
- back pain is often chronic with acute exacerbations
- symptoms are often non-specific
- it may be a warning sign of extremely serious pathology
- some, less scrupulous, patients are aware of diagnostic difficulties and may use back pain to malinger
- signs on examination may be absent or difficult to elicit.

A wrong diagnosis of malingering when the patient has metastatic prostate cancer will not be helpful to the patient or the GP! With these things in mind, care in history taking is paramount and the examiner will closely observe the thoroughness of the candidate's approach.

80

Specific of a history of back pain

Pain

Site.   The patient may use odd terms like 'lumbago'[13] and sciatica[14] when describing the pain. Make sure you understand what the patient means. The most common site is lumbar and if due to root irritation or compression may also cause spasm, which is frequently described as a generalised spasm.

Severity. Important for many reasons. The pain may be very severe and debilitating, preventing the performance of even the simplest of tasks. Paradoxically, back pain due to malignancy may often be vague and cause no incapacity.

Timing.   Malignant pain tends to be worse on waking whilst mechanical pain tends to be worse following activity.

---

[13] Origin from Latin, lumbus = loin
[14] Origin from Latin, Inschiadicus = hip

Table 3.6

Pathological origin	Mechanism of injury	Exacerbating features
Muscular strain	Flexion	Flexion/twisting
Disc herniation	Flexion/compression	Flexion/sitting
Facet joint	Extension/rotation	Extension/rotation
Sacroiliac joint	Fall onto bottom	Walking/sitting
Nerve root irritation	Flexion/compression	Flexion/sitting

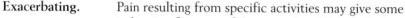

LOCOMOTOR

Exacerbating.	Pain resulting from specific activities may give some indication **features** of diagnosis (see Table 3.6). Pain on defecation, rising from a standing position, getting out of bed, etc., may point to nerve-root pathology, whilst localised pain on walking favours a bony cause.
Relieving factors.	Inflammatory pain may be relieved by NSAIDs. Mechanical pain may be relieved by rest, lying down or stretching.
Change in severity.	Most acute episodes of back pain (maybe as many as 80%) will resolve within 6 weeks of onset. Deteriorating pain may indicate more serious pathology.
Onset.	Slow or rapid, was there any associated trauma, direct injury or twisting?

Associated symptoms

Given that a recent onset of back pain may indicate one of a number of more serious diseases, a knowledge of these is critical for a safe and accurate diagnosis. Several signs and symptoms should alert you immediately to these causes and they must be assessed each time you take a history from a patient with low back pain. They are:

81

- **Progressive neurological deficit/urinary retention.** May be due to cauda equina compression. Ask about paraesthesia, shooting pains, pain in the distribution of the sciatic nerve, weakness, gait changes and bladder function. The sciatic nerve is the largest nerve in the body (L4, 5, S1–3) (Figure 7). Damage to the sciatic nerve itself may cause paralysis of the hamstring muscles and most of the muscles of the leg and foot but the 'sciatica' associated with nerve-root compression tends to follow the distribution of the compressed nerve root rather than the entire nerve. For example, pain in the distribution of the sciatic nerve and the dorsum of the foot, together with weakness of dorsiflexion of the great toe, suggests L5 root compression, whilst sciatic pain radiating to the lateral aspect of the foot with weak ankle plantar flexion is more likely if the S1 root is compressed.

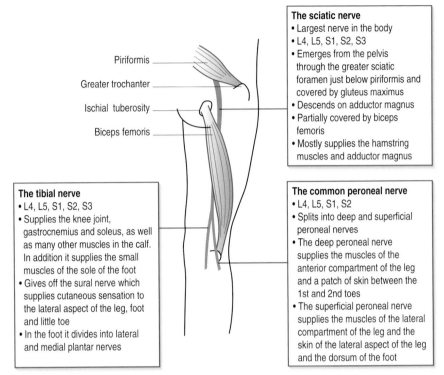

The sciatic nerve
- Largest nerve in the body
- L4, L5, S1, S2, S3
- Emerges from the pelvis through the greater sciatic foramen just below piriformis and covered by gluteus maximus
- Descends on adductor magnus
- Partially covered by biceps femoris
- Mostly supplies the hamstring muscles and adductor magnus

Piriformis

Greater trochanter

Ischial tuberosity

Biceps femoris

The tibial nerve
- L4, L5, S1, S2, S3
- Supplies the knee joint, gastrocnemius and soleus, as well as many other muscles in the calf. In addition it supplies the small muscles of the sole of the foot
- Gives off the sural nerve which supplies cutaneous sensation to the lateral aspect of the leg, foot and little toe
- In the foot it divides into lateral and medial plantar nerves

The common peroneal nerve
- L4, L5, S1, S2
- Splits into deep and superficial peroneal nerves
- The deep peroneal nerve supplies the muscles of the anterior compartment of the leg and a patch of skin between the 1st and 2nd toes
- The superficial peroneal nerve supplies the muscles of the lateral compartment of the leg and the skin of the lateral aspect of the leg and the dorsum of the foot

Figure 7 Schematic diagram of the right sciatic nerve in the lower limb

- **Back pain with pyrexia/fever.** Mechanical back problems are not normally associated with pyrexia. If the patient has back pain with a fever you should consider:
  - discitis: a disc space inflammatory condition thought to be due to infection. More common in children than adults, the pain is often very severe and localised to the affected disc. Patients with discitis tend to be lethargic and pyrexial.
  - spinal abscess: most commonly occur in the epidural space and may be secondary to infection elsewhere, although 30% have no obvious underlying cause. Perhaps surprisingly the pain is very often mild, but gradually gets more severe. There may be a sudden onset of neurological deficit. Intravenous drug use and diabetes are recognised risk factors.

Back pain in elderly people

The evaluation and management of back pain in older patients can be more difficult and complicated than in younger patients. There is a much wider range of possible diagnoses, including a much higher incidence of malignant causes.

When assessing an older person with back pain you must try to differentiate common musculoskeletal pain from serious visceral or non-spinal pain, and identify patients with primary nerve root pain; comorbidities; and complicating psychosocial issues. Musculoskeletal pain is likely to be due to vertebral fracture secondary to osteoporosis, so remember to ask about other fractures.

Back pain and cancer

Remember the six tumours that commonly metastasise to bone (see Box 3.5). Ask about general symptoms of malignancy, such as weight loss, anorexia, night sweats, etc.

Visceral causes of back pain

Remember that many abdominal diseases can be associated or even present with back pain. Abdominal aortic aneurysms and pancreatitis can present with acute or chronic back pain, as can cholecystitis and ovarian disease. Ask about associated abdominal pain and episodes of collapse.

A cautionary word

It is always worth looking for evidence of 'secondary gain' when assessing a patient with low-back pain. If the injury occurred at work, or you suspect that symptoms are subject to psychological overlay, you should make a careful record. **Do not,** however, presume that a patient is malingering until all other diagnostic possibilities have been eliminated and you have evidence of 'secondary gain' (i.e. do not make the diagnosis on the basis that you cannot fit the history and physical signs to another diagnosis).

Station extension

The examiner may show you an MRI scan or a plain radiograph of the spine and you must be familiar with both these investigations. Plain X-rays of the spine are very often normal even in patients with severe nerve root

---

Box 3.5 Cancers commonly metastasising to bone

Breast

Prostate

Kidney

Lung

Bowel

Thyroid

LOCOMOTOR

compression, but if shown a plain radiograph, you should look for a reduction in lumbar disc space and any associated signs of osteoporosis or osteoarthritis.

MRI scans give excellent anatomical pictures of lumbar discs and associated nerve root compression. However, they can be difficult to interpret and abnormalities can be subtle.

Suggestions for further practice

- **Primary care:** acute and chronic back pain is common. It is estimated to be responsible for the loss of 13 million working days in the UK each year and in excess of 1 in 10 primary care consultations are for back pain. The vast majority of low-back pain resolves with conservative or no intervention. It is not surprising that general practitioners are highly skilled in the diagnosis and management of back conditions. You should attend as many GP clinics as you can.
- **Orthopaedic clinics:** chronic back pain sufferers unresponsive to short-term conservative management are often referred to orthopaedic clinics. Most large hospitals now have orthopaedic surgeons who have a special interest in back disease.
- **MRI lists:** a true understanding of back problems means that you must understand the underpinning surgical anatomy of the back. MRI scanners offer a unique insight into the 'living anatomy' of the back.

Examination skills

OSCEs are a good method for assessing clinical examination skills. The short-station format allows examiners to test a wide range of examination skills rapidly and efficiently. In addition: they are:

- more objective, more reproducible and fairer than traditional short- and long-case clinical examinations
- the variability between examiners is reduced to a minimum
- all students are presented with the same test.

Despite the importance of history-taking skills in reaching a diagnosis, there are often more examination skills within an OSCE than history-taking stations. As there are only a limited number of systems/areas to examine (unlike history taking, where there are, potentially, an infinite number of variations on a theme), examiners tend to take a critical view of candidates who appear clumsy or unpractised whilst performing examinations. During the early years of the undergraduate programme, the examiners tend to focus on examination technique and ask the central questions:

- does the candidate look as though he has practised the skill?
- if so, is the candidate likely to pick up any abnormal signs?

As the programme progresses (even more so in postgraduate examinations) the examiner's focus changes toward the accurate description of any abnormalities that are present on examination.

Strategy for learning (basic)

Most system examination stations are five or six minutes in length. Like the history-taking stations, it is necessary to be succinct and precise in your performance of each clinical examination. The good news is that surgical examination stations are limited in number (Box 4.1). The bad news is that because examination stations are limited, examiners tend to expect a good level of competence in skill performance early in the undergraduate years.

When developing and honing your surgical examination skills we would suggest the following:

1. Concentrate on one system at a time. If you have decided that your next goal is to become proficient at rectal examination, then practice it until you are sure you have got your technique right.
2. There is no substitute for practice. You **cannot** become proficient at examining by:

   - watching other people
   - reading books
   - watching videos
   - having done it only once or twice.

3. Watch an experienced clinician perform the examination several times. Time them and watch their eyes and hands. You will notice that very

---

Box 4.1 Surgical examination stations

Skin lumps and bumps

Abdomen

Neck

Peripheral vascular system

Breast

Male genitalia/groin swelling

Eye

Ear

Hip

Knee

Shoulder

Back

Hands

Rectum

---

little time is wasted between aspects of the examination and the clinician will **look** as though he or she has performed the examination a thousand times (which of course he or she has!). Compare what you have seen with somebody who is at your stage of learning and make a note of the differences, particularly the places at which the learner pauses to remember what to do next.

4. Take **every** opportunity to practice your techniques. Don't restrict yourself to chance patient encounters, but utilise any clinical skills labs that you have at your disposal and practice (the more socially acceptable examinations only!) on fellow students and flatmates.

5. This book has attempted to include summaries of all the core skills for the common surgical examinations. You can use the core skills boxes as an aide-memoir to your practice.

6. Try to acquire a 'training buddy' or clinical partner who can observe and comment on your techniques.

A word about the video camera

Over the last few years at our institution, we have been running remedial classes for students who have difficulties with OSCEs. We have tried several techniques to improve student performance including supervised practice, formal and informal feedback and group working. The most successful technique we have employed, however, simply involves videoing a student performing an OSCE station and showing them the tape immediately after they have completed it. The results are remarkable; students often doubling their scores on their second attempt after watching themselves. One imagines that when they first see themselves they have the same feeling as a leading actor when he watches himself perform at the premier of a box office disaster! We recommend therefore that you seek out some video equipment and watch yourself perform. It may be an awful experience at first, but you will quickly see your own weaknesses across the range, from the way you approach your introduction to the patient, through to the hesitations between palpation and percussion. Try it once, then analyse your performance by looking at the bits you do well and the bits that you could improve and then try it again. Look specifically for:

- your introduction (how you greet the 'patient', your body language and posture)
- do you look comfortable in the situation (are you restless, jittery or do you have any visible bad habits)?
- which words do you use? (are they understandable to both examiner and patient?)
- how 'slick' or well-practised do you look?
- are there inaccuracies in the way that you perform the examination? (have you missed a bit or did you auscultate before percussing?)
- how did you end the station?

You will be pleased at how quickly your performance improves.

Strategy for learning (advanced)

As you become more adept in the techniques for examination, you will focus more and more on the abnormal and normal features of each individual patient. Your OSCE performance will reflect this development in cognitive thinking and by the time you reach higher/more advanced assessments, a large part of the examination stations will assess your ability to find abnormalities and recognise what is normal as well as your ability to perform a visibly competent examination. The OSCE simply reflects your developing ability as a doctor. Stations which require the student to examine and make diagnoses are often longer and may be incorporated into 'double stations' or, more recently, OSLER[1] examinations. The principles remain the same: a good and well-practised technique is likely to lead to a demonstration of the physical findings and a sound, accurate diagnosis.

Advanced examination stations often finish with a description of findings or further questioning on the diagnosis and/or an appropriate management plan. Common questions may be:

1. What abnormalities did you find?
2. Given your findings what is the most likely diagnosis?

---

[1] An Objective Structured Long Examination Record: a modification of an OSCE station, which is similar to an old style 'long case'. All candidates are assessed on the same 10 or so items by the examiner over 20–30 minutes. This improves the reliability of the assessment compared to the old long case. Particular attention is paid to the process of history taking and communication skills

3. Can you give me a list of the differential diagnoses based on your findings?
4. How would you investigate this patient?
5. Discuss the management plan for this patient.

In addition, the examiner may have the results of a subsequent investigation performed on the patient, which he will show you; typically, a radiograph, barium study or angiogram.

Learning strategies for these, more advanced, OSCE stations can be more difficult than those for the more basic exam-technique type stations, but there are several things that you can do to help yourself. Given that OSCEs require that many students can sit the same examination at the same time, administrators require patients that:

1. have signs that are relatively common in a hospital setting or out-patient department
2. have stable signs
3. have conditions that do not cause excessive pain on repeated examination
4. have signs that are 'hard' enough to be detected by the borderline student. In other words the signs are likely to be relatively obvious.

Considering the surgical examination stations that are listed in Box 4.1 above, it is possible to focus one's mind on examination stations which are more or less likely to occur within an OSCE (Table 4.1).

Therefore, a useful learning strategy is to seek out as many patients as possible with the commonly occurring conditions and examine them as frequently as you can. In addition, with each condition, see if you can answer the standard questions 1–5 as listed above.

How are you judged? Demonstrating competence

Presuming that the examiner has to decide if you are unsatisfactory, competent or excellent in the demonstration of your exam technique, he will use the following criteria to judge you:

- Was the student polite, empathic and understanding at all times?
- Were each of the standard sections of the examination completed in order and correctly?
- Was the technique used in inspection, palpation, percussion and palpation well practised?
- Did the student look as though he had performed the examination many times before? Did the examination 'flow'?
- Did the student explain the steps to the examiner/patient as indicated in the instructions?
- Is the examiner confident that the student would pick up any detectable abnormalities that are present?
- Differential diagnosis, investigations and appropriate management.

Table 4.1 Frequently and infrequently encountered OSCE stations

Examination	Frequently occurring	Unlikely
SKIN LUMPS		
Cutaneous	Sebaceous cyst	
	Basal cell carcinoma	
	Squamous cell carcinoma	
	Melanoma (although normally a picture rather than a patient)	
	Lipoma	
Subcutaneous		
Abdominal examination	Hepatomegaly	Ovarian cyst
	Splenomegaly	Stomach/colonic carcinoma
	Stoma	Aortic aneurysm
	Surgical scars	Diverticular mass
	Abdominal herniae	Intestinal obstruction
		Appendix mass
Peripheral vascular system	Common femoral occlusive disease	Peripheral aneurysms Gangrene
	Distal arterial occlusive disease	
	Arterial ulcer	
	Venous ulcer	
	Carotid stenosis	
	Amputation	
	A-V fistula	
	Varicose veins	
Hip	Osteoarthritis	Slipped femoral epiphysis
	Joint replacement	Perthe's disease
	Surgical scars	Acute fractures
		Dislocation
		Hip dysplasia
Knee	Osteoarthritis	Acute inflammatory disease
	Baker's cysts	Reiter's syndrome
	Knee replacement	Fractures
	Rheumatoid arthritis	Acute ligament/meniscal injury
Hands	Rheumatoid arthritis	Splinter haemorrhage
	Osteoarthritis	Fractures
	Carpal tunnel syndrome	
	Ganglion	
	Dupuytren's contracture	
	Clubbing	
Shoulder	Osteoarthritis	Dislocation
	Post surgery	

Examination	Frequently occurring	Unlikely
Back	Post surgery	Acute lumbar disc prolapse
	Ankylosing spondylitis	
	Osteoarthritis	Sacroileitis
Feet	Hallux valgus	
	Ulcers	
Male genitalia	Inguinal hernia	Testicular torsion
	Hydrocele	Epididymo-orchitis
	Varicocele	Testicular cancer
	Absent testicle	Femoral hernia
Eye	Cataract	Acute trauma
	Chronic glaucoma	Acute glaucoma
	Post surgery	Retinal detachment
	Diabetic retinopathy	
Ear	Chronic otitis media/ glue ear	Acute otitis media/externa Cholesteatoma
	Chronic perforation	
Breast lump	Breast cancer	Acute infection
	Fibroadenoma	
	Cyst	
	Post surgery	

Most examiners will tell you that they are fairly sure very early on during an OSCE station about a student's competence/incompetence, illustrating that an overall aura of confidence and experience are vital in achieving good marks.

A word about role-play

If your medical school uses simulated patients (SPs) for teaching and examining, we would suggest that you spend some time observing them in action. Many schools rely on such professionals for teaching purposes. As this form of teaching grows in popularity, simulated patients have become more and more skilled at their craft. If you talk to a simulated patient they will tell you that one of the most difficult skills they need to learn is 'staying in role'. As they are assuming a character that is not their own, they struggle to prevent themselves slipping out of role. Some SPs spend many hours focusing on their role before playing the part to prevent such a thing from happening.

In many ways, students who are able to stay in role, and come in and out of role at will, perform the best in an OSCE setting. Unfortunately this is an art that is difficult to learn and you are not normally required to formally role-play in your day-to-day clinical experiences. Role-play, therefore, is an art that you have to learn **specifically** for an OSCE.

Rectum

Level:	*
Setting:	A pelvic male mannequin (see Figure 8)
Time:	5 minutes

Comment

It may seem odd that we have chosen to start this section on examination technique with the bottom end of the GI tract, and with an area that can only be examined during an OSCE by using a mannequin. However, as we shall see, this station illustrates so many of the unique aspects of an OSCE that the rectum is the natural place to start.

Task

E   This is Mr Jones. Would you demonstrate a rectal examination?
(Equipment provided: mannequin as illustrated, lubricant, disposable non-sterile gloves, tissue paper, and alcohol hand wash)

Comment

There are several immediate problems with this station that an astute observer may notice. These include:

- this is clearly NOT Mr Jones
- the mannequin is incomplete-having no torso, head or limbs

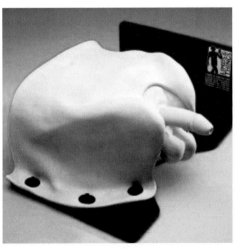

Figure 8 Typical rectal examination mannequin image. Courtesy of Limbs & Things

- the mannequin will not communicate
- there is a large piece of metal attached to the mannequin
- the setting is quite different from that which is usual for such an examination.

This sort of station is a particular favourite in OSCE examinations because the student can be assessed in core skills that may be difficult to assess in any other format. Examinations that are considered intimate can be assessed by using synthetic models, whereas real patients would be reluctant to undergo a rectal examination every 5 minutes for 3 hours! Unfortunately, the scenario will always be artificial to a greater or lesser extent and coping with these artificial environments is a core skill, central and specific to, a successful OSCE.

Core skill	Rectal examination

1. Seek a chaperone
2. Obtain verbal consent
3. Give clear instructions during the examination
4. Inspect the anus and surrounding areas
5. Prepare the gloved finger with lubricant
6. Insert the finger through the rectum using a posterior approach
7. Rotate the hand to examine the prostate and rectal wall
8. Wipe the anus with the gauze at the end of the examination

Starting the station

So you are faced with this station and your immediate thought is how 'silly' the scenario is. It is wise to take a few seconds to imagine the 'real' Mr Jones. You hold your hand out and introduce yourself and imagine Mr Jones shaking your hand back. You are now in role and the good candidate will stay in this role until the station ends. This technique of imagining the scenario within a true clinical setting will help in all stations involving mannequins. A suggested opening therefore, would be:

S   Good afternoon Mr Jones. My name is John Smith and I am a medical student. I have been asked to come and examine your back passage. Would that be OK?

P   *No response (or examiner responds).*

S   Thank you Mr Jones. Have you had this examination before?

P   *No response.*

S   Don't worry Mr Jones, I'll tell you exactly what I'm going to do step by step. It may be mildly uncomfortable but it should not be painful. If it is painful at any time then I will stop.

An average student will have learned this opening gambit and practiced it many times before. A good student will actually be imagining he is having a dialogue with Mr Jones and that the patient has responded at all points. In some OSCE stations like this, the examiner is instructed to verbally respond as though he/she was the patient. This can be either helpful or distracting, but the good candidate will be immersed in the scenario and respond to the examiner as though he/she were the patient.

Use of a chaperone

In a true clinical setting, there are occasions where chaperones are unavailable. For intimate examinations, like a rectal examination, a chaperone is essential and for most other examinations, desirable. In an OSCE session, requesting a chaperone **should be routine.** Here we meet a problem that hinders all role-play stations; how do we best ask for a chaperone? Most candidates will turn round to the examiner and say:

S (to the examiner) At this point I would obtain a chaperone.

In turning to the examiner the student has, by definition, come out of role. A professional simulated patient will tell you that jumping in and out of role like this is difficult and sometimes impossible, so how can you manage the problem? How about this:

S (to mannequin) If you just give me a second Mr Jones I'll just go and get a nurse to help me.

With this statement the student has:

- demonstrated to the examiner that he understands the importance of a chaperone
- stayed in role.

This principle of staying in role and playing out an OSCE station is central to achieving the highest possible marks.

The examination continues.

The principle of role-play as illustrated is demonstrated below in two ways. Firstly, by jumping in and out of role, and in the second example, the candidate attempts to stay in role. Try both methods and see which you feel most comfortable with; you may also want to video yourself doing this. Put yourself in the position of the examiner and ask yourself which of the answers you would give the highest marks for:

Answer 1: Jumping roles

Following the introduction, the student continues:

S (To examiner) I am now going to turn Mr Jones onto his left side (student rotates mannequin so buttocks facing him).

S (Puts gloves on, gets lubricant ready).

S (Student places hand on left buttock pulling buttocks gently apart). (To examiner) On inspection of the anal margin, I can see no scratching, thrombosed external piles, skin tags, fistulae or fissures.

S (Student puts drop of lubricant on gloved index finger, forefinger tip placed on anterior margin and with steady pressure finger slides into anus). (To mannequin) I'd like you to take some deep breaths through your mouth Mr Jones. (To examiner) The rectum is empty; the lateral and posterior walls are smooth. The prostate is smooth, of normal size and the sulcus is central. I can feel no masses.

S (Student gently withdraws finger and inspects the gloved index finger). (To examiner) There are no faeces and no sign of blood.

S (To mannequin) Thank you very much Mr Jones (wipes anus with gauze and turns mannequin onto back).

S Student washes hands with alcohol hand wash provided.

Station ends (time taken by the student approximately 3 minutes).

Comment

The student has handled this station in textbook fashion and has performed all parts of the core skill. Clearly the student is competent at the examination and the examiner would have to award a pass. However, the examination has been fragmented by constant referral to the examiner and, thus, may not appear slick. In addition, it would have been very easy for this student to have got lost and out of sequence because of the constant referral away from the patient towards the examiner. With the changes of role, the examiner would have found it difficult to determine the student's empathy and understanding of what Mr Jones would have endured, during what is a rather intimate, uncomfortable procedure.

Answer 2: Staying in role

Following the introduction the student continues:

S Mr Jones I'd like you to turn on to your left side, bring your bottom out to the edge of the bed and bring your knees up to your chest (student moves mannequin to left lateral position)

S As I said this may be slightly uncomfortable, so if you feel any discomfort you must tell me straight away and I will stop (student puts gloves on).

S (To mannequin) The first thing I'm going to do is to have a good look round the outside of your bottom (lifts left buttock). You can tell a lot from looking but that looks fine to me; I can't see any lumps or tears or scratches.

S (To mannequin) I'm now going to put my finger inside. It often helps if you take some deep breaths at this point to help you relax (puts lubricant on gloved index finger). I'm going to do this very slowly; once again if you have any pain I will stop straight away (forefinger tip placed on anterior margin and with steady pressure finger slides into anus).

S Well I can't feel anything in there so far, it seems completely empty. I'm now going to feel the sides and the back of your rectum. That's good, they are completely fine.

S (To mannequin) You may not be aware of this, but one of the reasons we do this examination is to feel a little gland called the prostate. I'm now going to examine it (student rotates finger to anterior rectal wall). That's very good Mr Jones, it seems to be the right size and shape and I can't feel anything abnormal.

S (To mannequin) OK I'm now going to take my finger out slowly. Once again would you take some deep breaths (student withdraws finger and visibly inspects gloved index finger). That seems to be normal.

S I'll just give you a little wipe and then you can turn onto your back again (student removes glove and disposes in bin, washes hands and returns mannequin to starting position, covering mannequin with blanket or sheet if available).

S Thank you very much Mr Jones. You have been very helpful.

Station ends (time taken by student approximately 4½ minutes).

Comment

When you first read answer 2, it may seem contrived, almost embarrassing. On further analysis, however, the student has performed excellently. Without coming out of role, he has completed the entire core skill whilst showing empathy and understanding for the patient. Both candidates (answers 1 and 2) have performed well and both would score an excellent mark. We advise that you attempt this station staying in and coming out of role so that you can find out which of the two methods suits you the best.

Level: *

Setting: A patient with a skin lump

Time: 5 minutes

Comment

Skin lumps are exceptionally common examination material. They are often
multiple and test the candidate's ability to **describe** what they see in an
organised, professional way. They very rarely involve role play, as most of
the lesions are so common that it is relatively easy to find willing patients to
participate in student doctor's education. In our companion book, *Core Clinical
Skills for OSCEs in Medicine*, there is a chapter on examination of the skin.
This focuses on global and regional skin changes such as a rash. Examining a
lump is very different and is very much a surgically orientated removal because
treatment most often requires operative removal of the lump.

Task

E   This gentleman has a lump (examiner points to the lump). Please examine it and
describe your findings to me.

Comment

The first thing you will notice is how specific the instructions are. You are told
specifically to identify the lump without recourse to a systems examination. It
follows that most marks will be awarded for the direct description of the lump,
not incidental findings or observations about the patient in general. Although
the examiner will expect you to be courteous to the patient and ask him/her
if you can examine the lump making reference to pain, this station does not
require you to pretend that you are within a normal clinical setting.

97

Procedure
Inspection

Inspection is a very important part of any examination. When examining a
lump, observation is very often critical in diagnosis. Because students are eager
to show that they know where to put their hands during an examination, or that
they know how to use a stethoscope, inspection is often glossed over. **Try to
take your time!**

It is a perfectly acceptable approach during this station to talk as you go along.
The examiner expects you to present your findings as you find them. Try to
learn a system for inspecting every lump such as:

GENERAL

- **Site:** describe it in as anatomically correct fashion as possible
- **Shape:** round, irregular, domed (try to describe it in three-dimensional terms)
- **Size:** it's a good idea to carry a small plastic ruler
- **Surface:** smooth, irregular/nodular
- **Shade (colour):** skin coloured, pigmented, light, dark
- **Multiple:** are the lesions multiple or solitary
- **Margin:** raised or flat, irregular or smooth; is the lesion discreet or does it blend into the surrounding skin
- **Palpation:** once again you can choose to talk as you examine or complete palpation and present your findings
- **Warmth:** examine with the back of your hand
- **Consistency:** soft, firm, hard, rubbery, stony
- **Fluctuence:** for lumps > 2 cm. Use three finger test
- **Edges:** are they well or poorly defined
- **Pulsatility:** is there a thrill?
- **Expansile:**
- **Transilluminable:** always carry a pen torch
- **Fixation:** does the skin move over the lump or is it embedded within? Is it fixed to any neighbouring structures?
- **Cough impulse**
- **Reducibility**
- **Percussion/auscultation:** percussion is rarely necessary for skin lumps and auscultation required only when you suspect the lesion is vascular when you should listen for a thrill.

S I would now like to examine the regional lymph nodes.

It is probably better that you state this at the end of the station and wait for the examiner's reaction. It is likely that the examiner will say that it is not necessary but regional-lymph-node examination is an **essential** part of the examination of any skin lump.

Common errors

Despite the apparent simplicity of this station, many students struggle. The commonest errors include those shown in Table 4.2.

Common skin lumps

In reality there are very few skin lumps that regularly appear in OSCEs (Table 4.1). However, as a very common follow-on question is the differential diagnosis, it is wise to think about this in relation to common skin lumps and include the rarer conditions. When asked about differential diagnosis, it is better to start with the most likely causes before launching into rarer ones. Try to make your list sensible. If, for example, you diagnose an obvious lipoma don't suggest that the main differential diagnosis is with a malignant melanoma; their characteristics are very different. A favourite line of questioning is:

Table 4.2 Common errors whilst examining a skin lump

Common errors	Learning strategy
Lack of familiarity with the descriptive features of a lump	**Learn a system for lumps**
Too short a time spent on inspection	**Practice describing lumps from pictures in a book so you can't touch them**
Failure to transilluminate/look for fluctuence	**Get into the habit of attempting to transilluminate and test for fluctuence on all lumps that you see even if you know that neither test is likely to be positive. Always carry a pen torch**
Attempting to percuss and auscultate obvious minor skin lesions	**Use your common sense**
Failure to request examination of regional lymph nodes	**Get into the habit of always looking for regional lymphadenopathy**

E   What else might the lump be?

A weaker student will then go on to list all the potential diagnoses of any skin lump. What the examiner actually means is:

E   What else is the lump **likely** to be?

Table 4.3 below lists the common **likely** differential diagnoses with each of the common skin lumps. Try to stick to these in your answer.

Station extension

These will depend on the diagnosis. With hernias, for example, the examiner may ask you about indications for surgery or even the basics of surgical repair. With skin lumps they may wish to talk about indications for excision.

Suggestions for further practice

Learn a system for describing all lumps. Break the system down into inspection and palpation. Skin lumps are very common and most patients with unrelated reasons for hospital admission will have several. Each time you come across a lump, try to describe it in your head or if you are with a colleague or teacher, describe it to them using the system you have learned.

GENERAL

Table 4.3 Differential diagnosis of skin lumps

Common diagnosis	Common differential diagnoses	Rare differential diagnoses
Sebaceous cyst	Lipoma Epidermal cyst Dermatofibroma	Gouty tophus Osteoma cutis Skin metastases Cylindroma
Lipoma	Sebaceous cyst Ganglion Lymph node	Soft tissue sarcoma Skin metastases
Lymph node	Sebaceous cyst Lipoma Skin abscess (if tender)	Soft tissue sarcoma Neurofibroma
Ganglion	Tenosynovitis Osteophyte Lipoma	Venous malformation Neuromas Hamartoma Sarcoma
Melanoma	Naevus Dermatofibroma Campbell de Morgan spots (angiokeratoma) Seborrhoeic keratosis	Accessory nipple Haemangioma Pigmented basal cell carcinoma Tinea nigra Verruca vulgaris
Basal cell carcinoma	Keratoacanthoma Seborrhoeic keratosis Nummular eczema Lichen planus Psoriasis	Amelanotic melanoma Paget's disease
Squamous cell carcinoma	Bowen's disease (in situ squamous cell carcinoma) Dermatitis Psoriasis Keratoacanthoma	

Legs (vascular arterial)

Level: **

Setting: A patient with intermittent claudication

Time: 5–10 minutes

Task

E   This patient is complaining of pain in his legs on walking 100 yards. I want you to examine his peripheral vascular system and comment on your findings as you go along.

Response

A key element in this station is talking the examiner through your examination and findings. Comment on both normal and abnormal findings.

Expose the whole of the lower limbs from the groin to the feet. Make sure you don't miss or fail to comment on obvious abnormalities such as scars from arterial bypass surgery (e.g. femoro-popliteal bypass).

Inspection

Always look at the whole leg and foot, specifically check the heel and between the toes and the plantar surface of the foot (common sites of ischaemic ulceration).

Comment on:

Scars – Commonly groin, medial aspect of thigh and along great saphenous vein.

Ulceration – Describe the site and shapes of the ulcer/s. Arterial ulcers are usually punched out with little or no sign of healing and may be extremely tender, so be gentle. Venous ulcers are typically situated over the medial malleolus and may be associated with varicose veins and dry, thickened and pigmented skin (venous eczema).

Signs of gangrene – It would be extremely unusual to see gangrene in an OSCE, because it constitutes a surgical urgency; it is more common to see pre-gangrene. Purplish-looking skin and sometimes 'diabetic' toes, which are dusky and on occasions black.

Varicose veins – These are not related to arterial disease. If you see obvious varicose veins comment on them and explain to the examiner that they are best examined with the patient standing up. Also make it clear that you know they are not related to arterial disease.

101

CARDIOVASCULAR

Capillary return – Gently press the skin over the side of the great toe, a bony prominence (usually the first metatarso-phalangeal joint) or the toenail. It often helps to try more than one site. If you are unsure if capillary return is prolonged (usually <2 s), compare with the other side or the patient's finger.

Vascular angle – Slowly raise the leg with your hand under the heel and applying light pressure with the other hand to empty the veins. Pause every 10 degrees or so. In patients with moderate-to-severe peripheral vascular disease the skin will become pale and veins show guttering somewhere between 10 and 45° from the horizontal.

Skin changes – These are not reliable, but look for skin thinning and loss of hair. By the end of the inspection you should have a pretty good idea that there is reduced perfusion of the limb. This helps your confidence, as you are not then entirely reliant on your ability to feel the pulses.

Palpation

Examine the peripheral pulses:

- Femoral: halfway between the anterior superior iliac spine and the symphysis pubis.
- Popliteal: the knee should be flexed to about 90° with the foot resting on the bed. Place your fingers around the back of the knee in the popliteal fossa. The pulse is best felt by palpation against the back of the tibial plateau rather than in the apex of the popliteal fossa (classical teaching).
- Posterior tibial: one-third of the way between the medial malleolus and tip of the heel.
- Dorsalis pedis: about half way up the foot in the first metatarsal space, just lateral to the extensor hallucis longus tendon.

When commenting on pulses state whether the pulse is present or absent. Comparison with the other side is encouraged.

A simple grading system is:

0   = Absent

+   = Barely palpable

++   = Reduced

+++   = Normal

Examination of the pulses may tell you where the blockage is:

- Femoral absent: iliac or aortic
- Femoral present, popliteal absent: superficial femoral
- Femoral and popliteal present, distal absent: distal disease.

Comment on skin temperature changes using the back of your hand and moving up the limb:

Aorta. Abdominal palpation for aortic aneurysm is a routine part of the examination of the arterial vasculature of the lower limb. To avoid causing a patient unnecessary discomfort, we suggest that you comment to the examiner that you would now like to proceed to abdominal palpation. The examiner will indicate to you if she expects you to carry out such an examination.

Neurological examination. At the end of the examination you should turn to the examiner and suggest that you perform a neurological examination of the lower limbs. This would routinely be performed in diabetic patients with PVD.

Auscultation

Listen over the femoral artery and aorta for bruits. You can practice this on your femoral artery. Press your stethoscope over your femoral artery until you can hear the turbulent flow.

Extension to station (Level***)

The station could be changed in a number of ways. A volunteer with no abnormalities could be used to determine whether you can perform the basic examination. This could be linked to a photograph of a patient with gangrene, diabetic foot problems or an arteriograph. Make sure you can identity the aorta, iliac, femoral, popliteal, anterior and posterior tibial arteries on an arteriogram.

Suggestions for further practice

The vascular ward and particularly the vascular outpatient clinic are the ideal places to see these patients.

Legs (venous)

Level:	*
Setting:	A patient with varicose veins
Time:	5 minutes

Task

E Examine the lower limb venous system.

We have included this station to illustrate how a very simple task can easily be handled badly in the stressful OSCE environment. Varicose veins are exceptionally common; there are over 2.5 million people in the UK with the condition at any one time. Most of these people are well and many are young and robust, and are easily recruited for examinations. Despite seeing varicose veins many times, students handle varicose-vein OSCE stations badly. The reason for this appears to arise from an obsession with the Trendelenburg or tourniquet test. This is a test that is an integral part of the traditional examination of the peripheral, superficial venous system. It is complicated to master and can be confusing to understand. If it is performed badly, it makes the examinee look clumsy. When confronted with this task in an OSCE it is easy to be distracted by the thought of having to perform the test at the end of the examination. The subsequent anxiety can be distracting and it is not uncommon to see a student completely forget the basics of the examination and forget to inspect or palpate the limb in an orderly fashion. A subsequent attempt at the Trendelenburg test is doomed to failure because of shaking hands and anxiety.

Paradoxically, because of the increased use of handheld Doppler, the Trendelenburg/tourniquet test is virtually redundant in modern medicine. In an OSCE, at most, it will carry one mark, whilst the inspection and palpation aspects of the skill will carry the bulk of the marks. There are many examination techniques with similar tests (e.g. the Trendelenburg test in examination of the hip, or the McMurray test in examination of the knee).

To overcome these difficulties in all OSCEs the following should be remembered:

- The bulk of marks in an examination station are ALWAYS awarded for the basics: inspection, palpation, percussion (fewer marks) and auscultation.
- Practice specific tests until you are competent.
- It is unlikely to be a matter of failure if you make a mistake with a single complicated test.

| Core skill | Examination of lower limb venous system |

1. Introduction and explanation
2. Expose both limbs to the groin
3. Stand the patient up and look at both limbs in turn. Look specifically for anatomical distribution of varicose veins, scars and ulcers (look specifically on the dorsum of the foot, above the medial malleolus and between the toes)*
4. Palpate the abnormal veins. Compare both sides, as they are often different anatomically and pathologically. Look for tenderness and thrombosis. Look around the ankle for dermatoliposclerosis or pitting oedema
5. Specifically palpate for the saphenofemoral junction (2–3 cm below and lateral to the pubic tubercle). Ask the patient to cough
6. Ask the patient to cough whilst palpating the popliteal fossa
7. Tap test
8. Trendelenburg/tourniquet test
9. Say: 'I would now like to examine the abdomen and do a rectal examination and either a scrotal or pelvic examination'

* Although varicose ulcers tend to occur in the lower area of the leg and particularly above the medial malleolus, the examiner will expect you to be able to differentiate between arterial and venous ulceration

Saphena Varix

This is a dilatation of the long saphenous vein in the groin just before it enters the femoral vein. It is caused by an incompetent valve at the saphenofemoral junction. The varix may be visible and palpable by the patient or picked up during an examination for varicose veins. Characteristically, it empties on compression and produces a fluid thrill when percussed. They are often delicate and can burst spontaneously or during varicose-vein surgery.

Tap test

In this test the fingers are placed at the distal end of one of the larger varicose veins. The top end of the vein is tapped with the fingers of the other hand and if there is an intervening incompetent valve you should feel a percussion impulse. This is a highly subjective test and of little value, but continues to be described in most surgical textbooks. It is unlikely to carry many marks, if any, in an OSCE station.

Trendelenburg/Tourniquet test

Both of these tests attempt to locate the site of venous incompetence. The tourniquet test is a modification of the Trendelenburg test. Strictly speaking the Trendelenburg test should be called the Brodie[2]–Trendelenburg test to differentiate it from the Trendelenburg test for hip stability.

The patient is asked to lie flat and one leg is elevated until the superficial veins are emptied by gravity. Two fingers are placed firmly at the saphenofemoral junction and the patient is asked to stand up whilst pressure is kept over the junction. The leg is observed for venous filling. If the only incompetent valve is the one at the saphenofemoral junction then the long saphenous vein will fail to refill and stay collapsed. If the vein fills then there must be valvular incompetence below the junction.

The tourniquet test utilises the same principle, but in this test the tourniquet is initially applied around the limb just below the saphenofemoral junction. The test is repeated moving the tourniquet down the limb 10 cm at a time until the veins below the limb fill. In this way the site of incompetence can be determined. As a rule of thumb, the tourniquet test only needs to be performed if the Trendelenburg test does not reveal saphenofemoral incompetence. The authors recommend that you suggest to the examiner that you would like to do the test before embarking upon it as the examiner is unlikely to want you to proceed because of time constraints.

Follow-up questions

You are likely to be asked about the following:

- **The causes of varicose veins:** Studies have suggested that female sex, increased age, pregnancy, geographical site and race are risk factors for varicose veins; there is no hard evidence, despite popular belief, that family history or occupation are factors. Obesity does not appear to carry any excess risk.
- **Indications for surgery:** Lipodermatosclerosis leading to venous ulceration, bleeding saphena varix and recurrent thrombosis are the principal indications for surgery, but most surgery is carried out for cosmetic reasons.
- **Investigations you might perform:** Fitness for anaesthesia should be assessed. In addition, Doppler scanning has become the investigation of choice for isolating incompetent valves.

---

[2] Sir Benjamin Collins Brodie (1783–1862) English Surgeon

Male genitalia

Level: *

Setting: A male pelvis mannequin on a table

Time: 5 minutes

Scenario

E This is Mr Jones (pointing to a male mannequin). I would like you to show me how you would examine his external genitalia.

Comment

The reason for including this station is that it is frequently badly handled by students. Nine times out of ten this is because of a lack of clinical experience in examining this area. Prior to OSCEs, it was rarely asked, even in postgraduate exams, because of the difficulty in getting male patients to participate. Modern-day mannequins, however, are very lifelike and of good quality. Thus, this is an increasingly common task.

Getting clinical experience in this area may be difficult, but it is essential that you seek out every opportunity. Many students find that attendance at several genito-urinary or urology outpatient clinics is extremely useful.

An additional difficulty can arise when students are unfamiliar with the types of mannequin available for this examination. Try to become as familiar as you can with the resources available in your own clinical skills unit.

Core skill	Examination of the male genitalia

1. If asked – talk to the model or examiner (role play as far as you can)
2. Obtain clear consent
3. Inspection – ulcers/lesions around the penis and scrotum, mucosal ulceration, and urethral discharge. Retract foreskin and inspect glans
4. Note whether the left testis is slightly lower. Palpate each testis and vas deferens, and comment on its presence, shape, size, consistency, swellings, asymmetry and any associated masses
5. Trans-illuminate any swellings
6. Examine local lymph nodes
7. Finish by saying you would examine, abdomen, groins and rectum

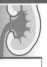

Inspection

1. Always use gloves
2. Look at the skin for any obvious scars, lumps or ulcers
3. Retract the foreskin to detect any chancres or friable masses (carcinoma of the penis in the early stages is frequently obscured by the foreskin)
4. The presence of cheesy white material accumulating under the foreskin (smegma) is a sign of poor personal hygiene
5. Is the foreskin difficult to retract (phimosis)?
6. Look at the glans for ulcers or inflammation (balanitis)
7. Look at the base of the penis for any excoriations
8. Study the urethral meatus. Is it in the right place? Is it displaced to the inferior surface (hypospadias)? Is it displaced to the upper surface (epispadias)?
9. Look for urethral discharge by compressing the glans between the thumb and index finger:
   - profuse and yellow = gonococcal urethritis
   - scanty, white or clear = non-gonococcal urethritis.

Palpation

1. Palpate the shaft of the penis between thumb and first two fingers of your right hand
2. If the prepuce is retracted, replace it
3. Feel for any plaques, thickening or tight bands/scarring
4. Carefully palpate testis and scrotum. Feel for the epididymis and the body of the testis. Gently feel for the spermatic cord
5. Palpate the inguinal lymph nodes.

Transillumination

Use a pen torch to shine a light from behind any testicular mass that you find.

Comment

Examining the male genitalia does not take a long time; therefore the examiner will almost always be armed with supplementary questions for you once you have finished. Be familiar with the common disorders (Table 4.4).

Extension to station (Level***)

A thorough examination of the male genitalia may be performed in just a few minutes. It is not uncommon for such a station to include a picture such as the one in Figure 9. The examiner may ask you to comment on the test being performed, the abnormality shown or the relevant clinical anatomy. Most surgical atlases will have multiple examples of scrotal and penile abnormalities. These atlases can be a useful adjunct to your own clinical experience.

Table 4.4 Common disorders of the male genitalia

Common disorders of the male genitalia	Clinical findings
Penis	
Syphilitic chancre	Dark, red painless ulcer
Genital herpes	Cluster of small vesicles and shallow non-painful ulcers with red bases
Venereal warts	Often moist and malodorous friable masses
Carcinoma of the penis	Indurated, non-tender nodule or ulcer
Scrotum	
Varicocele	Easily distinguishable from the testis, often does not feel like the classical 'bag of worms'
Hydrocele	Non-tender fluid-filled mass, transilluminates and you can normally 'get above it'
Spermatocele	Painless mobile cystic mass just above the testis
Testicular cancer	Painless hard nodule on testis
Epididymitis/acute orchitis	Tender, swollen epididymis. Scrotum may be red and swollen. Inflamed, tender, swollen testis
Testicular torsion	Acutely tender painful and swollen: a surgical emergency!

If you are examining a real patient and detect a **scrotal swelling**, then consider four questions:

Question 1: Can I get above the swelling?

- No – it is an inguinal hernia
- Yes – it is a primary scrotal swelling.

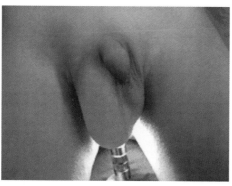

Figure 9 A scrotal swelling in a 5-year-old child

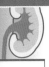

Question 2: Is it cystic?

- Testis and epididymis felt separately – epididymal cyst. The cyst is usually felt just above the testis
- Testis and epididymis not felt separately and testis difficult to feel – hydrocele (most will transilluminate).

Question 3: Is it solid?

- Arising in the testicle – most likely to be a tumour. Tumours are sometimes associated with a lax hydrocele
- Arising in the epididymis – most likely to be a small epididymal cyst or thickened epididymis secondary to infection.
- A varicocele is easily distinguished from the testicle and may feel like the classic description of a 'bag of worms', though this is not always the case.

Question 4: Is the testis tender?

- If palpated too hard even the normal testis will be tender
- Most tumours are painless and non-tender
- A patient with epididymo-orchitis usually has an exquisitely tender testis.

Suggestions for further practice

The authors strongly recommend that you repeatedly revisit the anatomy of the male genitalia throughout your clinical studies. It is an embryologically complicated area that freque ntly forms the basis of clinical examination questions in general surgery. It is insufficient to learn the anatomy from a book or atlas alone as it can only be appreciated if observed in a three-dimensional environment such as the dissecting room or in theatre. Many medical schools now have joint tutorials between anatomists and surgeons to bring the anatomy and pathology of such areas alive for the learner. If your institution has such events you are strongly advised to attend.

Neck

Level: ***

Setting: A 40-year-old female patient in a high-backed chair

Time: 5 minutes

Task

E This lady has a swelling in her neck. Can you see it?

S Yes, there is a bulge in the front of her neck slightly to one side.

E Before I ask you to examine this lady's neck, would you care to hazard a guess as to what is causing the swelling?

S Judging by the patient's age and the position and size of the lump, I think the most likely site is the thyroid.

E What other organs or tissues may cause a swelling in this area?

S Lesions in the skin, subcutaneous tissues and lymph nodes.

E OK. I'd now like you to examine this lady's neck fully.

Comment

Because of the anatomical and structural complexity of the neck, short OSCE stations tend to be accompanied by more specific instructions than just a general request to examine the neck. The key to neck examination, however, is inspection because any gross abnormality will not only be visible, but will also act as a pointer to where the examination will lead and hence how your examination technique should be tailored. For example, an enlarged thyroid would make you look for signs of hypo- or hyperthyroidism, a pulsatile carotid mass would lead you to focus on the arterial system whilst an enlarged parotid gland would lead you to examine the facial nerve.

Inspection (from the front)

Attention to detail is the order of the day when examining the neck. A structured practiced approach, taking time to consider the main anatomical areas is essential.

Take care to inspect:

- the skin
- the parotid region
- the anterior triangle including the sub-mandibular triangle

111

ANATOMY ESSENTIALS: **The neck**

1. When describing abnormalities, the neck is divided into posterior and anterior triangles by the sternocleidomastoid (SCM) muscle. (Palpate your own SCM by turning your chin towards your left shoulder and feel the right side of the neck.)

2. Most of the cervical nerve plexus emerges in the posterior triangle and the spinal accessory nerve (cranial nerve XI) runs from the posterior border of SCM across the posterior triangle to the anterior border of trapezius.

3. The anterior triangle contains:
   - carotid artery and jugular veins
   - hyoid bone and thyroid cartilage (forming the Adam's apple)
   - below the Adam's apple is the cricoid cartilage and the thyroid gland.

4. The thyroid gland lies on either side of the trachea and crosses it anteriorly at about the second cartilaginous ring. The thyroid is covered anteriorly by the thin strap muscles and lies in part under the SCM muscles.

- the anterior jugular area
- the posterior triangle.

Always ask the patient to take a sip of water. A thyroid mass will move upwards on swallowing. If you think that a mass may be of thyroid origin, ask the patient to stick their tongue out. This is helpful because a thyroglossal cyst (rare cause of thyroid/neck swelling) will move, because of its embryological origin, on tongue protrusion.

Palpation

The neck should be palpated from behind with the examiner standing and the patient seated. Explain this to the patient because you will be out of the patient's eye line and she may find this disconcerting. Use the same system for palpation as you used for inspection, making sure to examine the parotid, thyroid, anterior triangle, anterior jugular area and posterior triangle. Describe any mass that you find in the way that you would describe any abnormality elsewhere, focusing on shape, size, consistency, etc. If there is a palpable anterior mass, ask the patient to take another sip of water to see if it moves with swallowing.

Core skill   **Examination of the neck**

1. Introduce yourself and explain to the patient what you are going to do
2. Expose the neck completely down to the clavicles and prevent hair from obstructing your view
3. Look from all directions at the same level as the patient. If the patient is sitting, then either sit at her level or ask her to stand
4. Give the patient a glass of water and comment on what you see

GASTROINTESTINAL

5. Ask the patient to protrude their tongue and comment on what you see
6. Palpate the neck from behind. Comment on thyroid, thyroid masses and any other masses particularly lymphadenopathy
7. Whilst gently feeling the thyroid, ask the patient to take a further drink of water and ask them to protrude their tongue
8. Examine the supra-clavicular, infra-clavicular and occipital nodes
9. Auscultate for bruits over the thyroid and the common carotid bifurcation

Table 4.5 Swellings in the neck

Common	Benign lymphadenopathy	URTI
		Tuberculosis
		Viral pharyngitis
		HIV
		Glandular fever
	Malignant lymphadenopathy	Lymphoma
		Leukaemia
		Metastatic head and neck cancer
		Other malignancy
	Thyroid gland bilateral and diffuse	Inflammatory (Hashimoto's/de Quervain's)
		Anaplastic carcinoma
		Graves disease
	Thyroid gland bilateral and multi-nodular swelling	Multi-nodular goitre
	Thyroid gland unilateral and solitary swelling	Colloid cyst
		Adenoma
		Carcinoma (papillary/follicular)
Not as common	Salivary gland enlargement	Mumps
		Stone
		Tumour
		Bacterial infection
Rare	• Pharyngeal pouch	
	• Cervical rib	
	• Subclavian artery aneurysm	
	• Thyroglossal cyst	
	• Branchial cyst	
	• Chemodectoma	
	• Sternomastoid tumour	

113

The reason that we have graded this station as ··· is because the next part of the examination depends wholly on your findings on initial inspection or palpation. We will consider only those that are likely to arise in an OSCE.

Example 1: A Thyroid mass

Specifically look for:

- shape of the swelling
- midline or lateral
- unilateral or bilateral
- nodular or smooth
- multiple or single nodules
- movement with swallowing
- can you get above and below it (is it retrosternal)?

Following palpation of a thyroid mass, it should then be auscultated for bruits, which represent the hyperdynamic flow sometimes detectable in Grave's disease.

At this point, the examiner may prompt you:

E Is there anywhere else you would like to examine?

S Yes I would like to look for signs of hyper- or hypothyroidism.

E How would you look for signs of hyper- or hypothyroidism?

Hyperthyroid
- General cognition: anxious and jumpy
- Pulse: tachycardia, wide pulse pressure
- Skin: warmth, sweating, signs of weight loss, pre-tibial myxoedema
- Eyes: lid lag, lid retraction, conjunctival injection, exopthalmos, ocular muscle weakness
- Nervous system: hyper-reflexia, proximal myopathy.

Hypothyroid
- General cognition: slow to respond, anhedonic or depressed
- Skin: cool and dry
- Pulse: slow, low-volume pulse
- Hair: patchy alopecia or thinning
- Nervous system: delayed relaxation of reflexes.

Common supplementary questions
E How would you investigate the mass in the thyroid?

S I would perform blood tests including thyroid function tests. I would then arrange a chest radiograph including thoracic inlet views if there was a clinical suspicion of a retrosternal goitre as well as an ultrasound of the neck. I would arrange fine-needle aspiration cytology (FNAC) of the abnormal area.

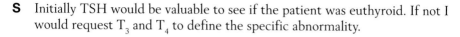

E   How would thyroid function tests help you?

S   Initially TSH would be valuable to see if the patient was euthyroid. If not I would request T$_3$ and T$_4$ to define the specific abnormality.

E   What are the limitations of thyroid ultrasound?

S   An ultrasound can help distinguish between solitary and multiple nodules. It can also accurately differentiate between cystic and solid lesions. It is not very sensitive or specific for thyroid malignancy however.

E   What are the benefits of FNAC?

S   Because there are several different diseases that can cause a thyroid swelling, a histopathological diagnosis is essential, so that the correct treatment can be undertaken. FNAC is currently the 'gold-standard' investigation for thyroid swellings. It is quick and can be reported immediately, it has a very low risk of tumour seeding and does not interfere with future surgery.

E   Do you know of any problems with FNAC?

S   It can cause bleeding and bruising and some thyroid diseases cannot be differentiated by FNAC alone. For example, it is difficult to tell the difference between benign and malignant follicular neoplasms with FNAC alone.

E   What type of thyroid cancers are you aware of?

S   The commonest type is papillary, which accounts for more than 70% of thyroid malignancies. There are also follicular, medullary and anaplastic types. Lymphomas can also occur in the thyroid.

115

Example 2: Cervical lymphadenopathy

Describe the shape and site of the nodes (see Figure 13 p 128). Are they hard or soft? Are there several nodes matted together or spaced some distance apart? Are they all in one chain, superficial cervical, deep cervical, occipital, sub-mental, sub-mandibular or are they in multiple chains? Are they hard or soft? Are they fixed to underlying structures or are they mobile?

E   Is there anywhere else you would like to examine?

S   Yes I would like to examine the remainder of the lymphatic system, the face, the breasts and inside the mouth. In addition I would also like to perform a general systemic examination, including all the major systems.

E   Why would you want to perform such an extensive additional examination?

S The lymph nodes can be enlarged in many diseases. Just because the first clinical presentation is a lymph node in the neck does not mean that any disease process is confined to the neck.

E How would you classify the underlying causes of cervical lymphadenopathy?

S I would initially divide the causes into infectious and non-infectious. The infectious causes can be localised, such as an upper-respiratory-tract viral infection, or systemic, like infectious mononucleosis. The non-infectious causes I would further divide into malignant and non-malignant. Metastases from oral, thyroid and other head and neck cancers are the most common, but lymphomas can present with enlarged neck lymph nodes as well. Non-malignant, non-infectious causes are rare, but things like sarcoidosis and psoriasis can cause lymph-node enlargement.

Comment

In order to adequately assess the lymphatic system of the neck you must have a basic understanding of the surface anatomy of the neck nodes. Be sure to revise this frequently as it is easy to forget some in the heat of the moment. The commonest cause of multiple cervical lymph-node enlargement is a viral upper-respiratory-tract illness. Solitary, firm lymph nodes greater than 2 cm in diameter, however, are more likely to have a more sinister origin.

Supplementary questions

E What investigations would you perform on a patient with a solitary 2 cm lymph node just anterior to the anterior border of sternocleidomastoid muscle?

S I would perform some basic blood tests including a full blood count and ESR. These may show evidence of an 'acute phase response' and would suggest the presence of systemic inflammatory disease. I would arrange a chest X-ray and arrange performance of a full examination of the nasopharynx including indirect laryngoscopy, to look for evidence of a primary malignancy. Depending on the results of these tests, more complicated investigations, such as a CT or MRI of the neck, may be necessary. It is important, however, to get an early histological diagnosis and early biopsy may be indicated if the initial investigations are not helpful in making a diagnosis.

E Often, in this situation, these tests come back negative. What would you do then?

S A definitive diagnosis could be obtained using fine-needle aspiration cytology, but if this were inconclusive, I would arrange an excision biopsy.

Abdomen

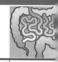

Level: */**

Subject: A simulated/real patient

Time: 5/10 minutes

Task

E Please show me how you would examine the patient's abdomen. I want you to describe what you are doing/looking for as you are going along.

Comment

This station is truly the 'bread and butter' of surgical examinations and it is surprising how often abdominal examination is done badly. Several common themes occur in students who do poorly at abdominal examination. These include:

- Not listening to the precise details in the instructions for the station (you may be asked to examine the abdomen, palpate the abdomen, etc.)
- Spending too long on inspection of the hands, face and eyes
- Uncertainty as to how much or little should be examined (groins, hernial orifices, lymph nodes, etc.)
- Excessive palpation that makes the patient uncomfortable
- Pausing to think about what to do next thus, lacking fluency or 'slickness'.

The common theme for all these problems is, once again, a lack of practice. Abdominal examination, to the surgeon, should be entirely routine. In addition, many of these problems can be avoided if you develop a quick rapport with the examiner who will tell you if you are doing too much or missing something, e.g:

S I would now like to examine the patient's groin and hernial orifices.

E Thank you but there is no need to do that on this occasion.

Inspection and patient positioning

S Hello, my name is John Smith, I'm a final-year medical student and I have been asked to examine your abdomen. Is that OK with you?

P *Yes that's fine.*

S May I ask your name?

P *Yes I'm David Carroll.*

S Mr Carroll, I'd first like to get you to lie as flat as you can, resting on just one pillow. Is that going to be uncomfortable for you?

P *No. That should be fine.*

Comment

Help the patient lie down. Most patients will require just one pillow on which to rest their head. The flatter the patient is, the greater the exposure of the abdomen. However, lack of relaxation in the neck muscles will cause the patient to tense their abdominal musculature making examination more difficult. Some elderly patients may require two or three pillows to feel comfortable. Observe for any signs of discomfort and act to avoid positions that you perceive as being uncomfortable.

Core skill	Abdominal examination

1. Inspection
   - General
   - Hands
   - Head and neck
   - Abdomen
2. Position the patient
3. Palpation
   - General
   - Liver
   - Spleen
   - Kidneys
4. Percussion
   - Shifting dullness
   - Liver
   - Bladder
5. Auscultation
6. Hernial orifices
7. Genitalia
8. Rectal examination

S I am going to have a little look at your hands and eyes.

Comment

At this point many surgeons will hold the patient's right hand as though they are shaking hands and at the same time gently feel the radial pulse with the left hand. When doing this ask yourself:

- Is the patient sweating?
- Are the hands warm?
- Is the pulse racing or slow?

Next hold the patient's hand with the palm facing you to look for signs of hyperaemia, palmar erythema or Dupuytren's contracture and then turn them

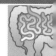

over to briefly look at the nail beds for clubbing, discoloration or lines in the nails themselves. Next, move to the sclera and look for jaundice. You will also observe that an experienced clinician may gently palpate the supra-clavicular and infra-clavicular fossae for lymphadenopathy. If you do this, make sure that you do not lose track of the central focus of the examination, and hands and eyes should take **no more than 30 s**. Practice on every patient you examine and time yourself.

Inspection

The tendency of most students is to spend too long on looking at the hands and face, and too little on inspecting the abdomen. The list of signs that can be seen simply by observation is vast and great care must be taken not to miss obvious or subtler abnormalities. Once you have positioned the patient flat with the hands down by the side, you must expose the abdomen. Traditionally an appropriate exposure is from nipple to groin but there are frequently practical problems. To avoid error in exposure turn to the examiner and state:

S I would usually expose the abdomen from the nipple (just below the breast in the female) to the groin.

The examiner will immediately respond with any limitations he feels are appropriate. As important as patient positioning is where you position yourself. Strictly speaking, symmetry should be assessed whilst looking along the midline, however, patients, particularly females, find it uncomfortable for a doctor to stand staring at their exposed abdomen from between their legs at the end of the bed. An appropriate compromise is to stand slightly to the side and well back. Explain at all times to the patient what you are doing to reduce this uncomfortable interaction.

In this scenario, the examiner has specifically instructed you to inform the patient what you are doing as you are going along. You must therefore describe your findings on inspection. The problem with any stressful scenario like an OSCE is the tendency to forget things easily. This can be avoided by practice, so that each step becomes second nature, and having a checklist of things you would specifically look for. For example:

- Abdominal movement. Is there movement on respiration, is the movement symmetrical? Ask the patient to blow their abdomen out and suck it in. Ask if this is painful. Any form of peritoneal irritation will make both these actions at best uncomfortable, at worst impossible. Look for signs of peristalsis. Finally, ask the patient to cough. Most herniae will be visible.
- Swelling. Is the abdomen distended? Is the swelling midline or localised to one side?
- Scars. Are there any obvious scars?
- Stomas. Are there any stomas? Where are they? Are they single-barrelled or double-barrelled? Is there an associated para-stomal hernia?
- Skin. Are there any marks/lesions on the skin?

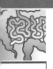

GASTROINTESTINAL

When mentally going through your checklist in this scenario, it is perfectly acceptable to mention negative findings. The examiner can then be sure that you are looking for the right things.

S On inspection the abdomen is moving normally with respiration. Mr Carroll is not showing any signs of discomfort. There is no obvious swelling. No visible masses, scars or herniae. There are no obvious skin changes.

Comment

It is not uncommon at this point for the examiner to interrupt and ask you to clarify what you can see or to ask a related question. Do not be distracted by this and be prepared. Common questions include:

- What operation may the patient have had? (appendicectomy, cholecystectomy, laparotomy, etc.)
- Where would you expect to see herniae on the abdominal wall? (groins, scars, etc.)
- What are the common causes of midline abdominal swelling? (obesity, flatus, pregnancy, bladder, etc.)

A word about scars and stomas

As you would imagine, most surgeons are interested in scars and, even if a scar is an incidental finding, most surgeons will be impressed with a student who identifies the scar and describes it correctly. In order to do this, you need to be familiar with the commonly occurring abdominal scars. The same is true of stomas. Figures 10 and 11 demonstrate the most commonly occurring stomas and scars. A typical description may sound like this:

S In the right upper-outer quadrant is a 15 cm oblique scar running 1 cm below the right costal margin. The scar is clean with no cross hatching. I think that it is called a Kocher's[3] incision and is a frequently used incision for exposing the gallbladder.

The surgeon could not help but be impressed!

In addition to the site of a scar, the scar itself can be abnormal. You should be aware that scars can be:

- atrophic (flat and white)
- hypertrophic (raised and reddened)
- keloid (raised, irregular and wide).

Palpation

S I am now going to gently feel your abdomen. Please tell me if it is uncomfortable at any stage and I will stop.

---

[3] Theodor Kocher (1841–1917) Swiss surgical polymath, Awarded Nobel Prize 1909

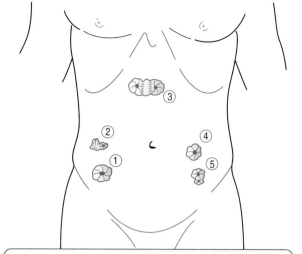

(1) Caecostomy (rarely used) or end ileostomy
(2) Defunctioning ileostomy (note two barrels, end ileostomy only has one)
(3) Transverse defunctioning loop colostomy (double barrelled)
(4) End colostomy
(5) Defunctioning colostomy (double barrelled)

Figure 10 Commonly occurring abdominal stoma sites

Comment

It is often said that the easiest way to fail a clinical examination is to hurt the patient. Although this is not strictly true, every effort should be made to consider the well-being of the patient, whether real or simulated. This is particularly true in an OSCE as you are unlikely to be the first or last student to examine that patient. Showing consideration will earn you respect and probably marks from the examiner. Get into the habit of kneeling down on the right side of the patient when palpating the abdomen. This action will bring your forearm and wrist into line and makes flexion of the MCP joints easier, making palpation itself more sensitive; in addition, standing over the patient whilst examining the abdomen can be intimidating. In clinical practice, it may not always be necessary, but it shows the examiner that you have the best approach to eliciting physical signs.

Palpation should be done systematically. Rub your hands together to make sure that they are not too cold (unlikely in the heat of an OSCE) and if they are, warn the patient. Starting in the left iliac fossa, gently palpate whilst keeping the fingers straight, bending them only at the metacarpo-phalangeal joints. As you are palpating all the quadrants of the abdomen, imagine the position of the colon and small bowel, and keep your eyes on the patient's face to make sure it is not too uncomfortable.

GASTROINTESTINAL

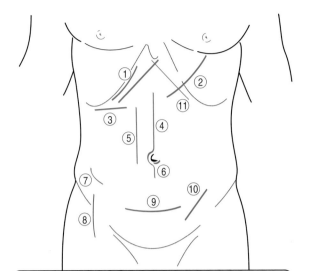

(1) Right hypochondrial (Kocher's incision)
(2) Thoraco-abdominal incision (normally for oesophagus)
(3) Transverse (mini-laparotomy for gallbladder)
(4) Midline (exploratory laparotomy)
(5) Paramedian (exploratory laparotomy, not commonly used today)
(6) Infra-umbilical (laparoscopic port site or umbilical hernia)
(7) Lanz (appendix)
(8) Vascular inguinal (access to femoral vessels)
(9) Transverse Pfannensteil (gynaecology)
(10) Inguinal (hernia)

Figure 11 Commonly occurring abdominal incisions

Once you have finished with gentle palpation and you are certain that the patient has felt no pain:

S I am now going to feel a bit deeper. Once again tell me if I am hurting you.

Repeat the process, this time feeling a bit deeper. Remember, keep looking at the patient's face. If it hurts at any stage acknowledge the discomfort.

S I'm sorry Mr Carroll. I'll try not to do that again.

The purpose of superficial palpation is to localise any discomfort and assess the patient's muscle tone for signs of peritonism, whilst deep palpation focuses on defining any gross abnormality, such as a mass.

Palpation of specific organs

Liver

Provided there is no pain, the liver may now be palpated. The liver itself enlarges towards the right iliac fossa. With the patient breathing slowly and deeply, place the flat of your hand in the right iliac fossa. Gradually move your

---

[4] Hermann Johannes Pfannenstiel (1862–) German Gynaecologist

ANATOMY ESSENTIALS: **The liver**

Think carefully about the surface anatomy of the liver; it is a large organ and fits snugly into the convex surface of the right hemi-diaphragm. Its upper border reaches to the level of the xiphisternal joint reaching the 5th intercostal space **on the left** 7–8 cm from the midline. On the right, it reaches the fifth rib at the front. The bulk of the liver is covered by the rib cage and, on normal shallow inspiration, it is usually not palpable at all.

hand in small increments, towards the right costal margin. Although there are a myriad of causes of an enlarged liver, by far the commonest in the UK are cardiac failure, metastatic carcinoma and the initial stages of cirrhosis (in the later stages of cirrhosis, the liver becomes shrunken). If you feel the edge of the liver, describe it like any other mass. Is it smooth or nodular, soft or hard? How much can you feel (normally measured in finger breadths or cm below the costal margin). Is it tender or painless?

Spleen

ANATOMY ESSENTIALS: **The spleen**

The spleen is impalpable in normal people. In fact it lies so high above the costal margin that it must be at least double its normal size before it can be felt. Remember the numbers 1, 3, 5, 7, 9 and 11. It measures 1 × 3 × 5 inches (2.5 × 7 × 12 cm) weighs 7 oz (just over 200 g) and lies between the 9th and 11th ribs. The spleen, like the liver, descends towards the right iliac fossa when it enlarges.

Start by palpating in the right iliac fossa and ask the patient to take some slow deep breaths through their mouth. Move the hand gradually up towards the left costal margin. Three techniques may help you identify a spleen that is just palpable:

1. Ask the patient to draw up their knees and relax their abdominal muscles
2. Lie the patient on their right side facing you and ask them to draw their knees up
3. Get the patient to lie back on your left hand and push the rib cage towards you whilst palpating for the spleen with your right hand.

Kidneys

This part of the examination confuses most students when they are learning abdominal examination and it takes practice to become proficient. The critical thing is to make sure that the patient relaxes. It is a bimanual technique and involves one hand pushing the kidney towards the other. A grossly enlarged kidney can be directly palpated in the loin. Smaller renal masses can be palpated by balloting the kidney (a ballot is a small ball). One hand is placed anteriorly in the loin and the other posteriorly. One hand is pressed towards the other; the renal mass is pushed forward and can be felt.

Percussion

Percussion should be firstly used as a confirmation of what you have found during palpation. Thus, the liver, spleen and any abdominal masses should be percussed. When percussing the liver start at the fourth intercostal space to avoid missing the upper border. Always start with the finger used for percussion on the abdomen parallel to the direction of the anticipated note change.

Core skill	Abdominal percussion

1. Percuss over any mass you find
2. Liver: start at 5th rib from the top or right iliac fossa from the bottom, keeping your fingers parallel to the costal margin
3. Spleen: start at RIF moving towards left hypochondrium
4. Shifting dullness

A word about percussing for ascites

For many years percussion for ascites was considered a gold-standard, clinical examination technique for the diagnosis of ascites. Several recently published studies have shown marked inter-observer errors when percussing for ascites and less emphasis is placed on it now. The reason for mentioning it here is that many students get bogged down worrying about their percussion technique. The authors suggest that you learn a quick technique which you can reproduce and cease worrying if you will 'pick up' ascites in an OSCE. We suggest the following technique:

1. Percuss from the umbilicus laterally (with your fingers pointing towards the head) and ascertain that the percussion note is resonant at the umbilicus (gas at the apex) and dull in the flanks (fluid-dependent). If this is not the case, then the patient does not have ascites.
2. Ask the patient to roll over towards you (on their right side), whilst keeping your hand over the left flank where it is dull. Wait for approximately 30 s then percuss again. The fluid should drain towards you, and the gas rise towards the left flank. Percuss again over your fingers – the note should now be resonant.
3. Keep your hand in the same position and ask the patient to lie on their back again and check if the original percussion note has returned.
4. The process can be repeated by rolling the patient onto their left side.

Auscultation

Abdominal auscultation should be simple. Bowel sounds should occur every 10–15s during normal peristalsis, but cannot be considered to be 'absent' until you have listened for a full minute. Bowel sounds are heard just below and lateral to the umbilicus.

Bowel sounds are either present or absent. If present, they are normal or abnormal in character. They are abnormal in character in intestinal obstruction when they are high-pitched or 'tinkling' and often loud. Increased frequency of bowel sounds may also be heard in infectious enteritis.

Finally, place the stethoscope just below and lateral to the xiphoid process to listen for arterial bruits.

Finishing the abdominal examination

Without being prompted turn to the examiner and say:

S I would now like to examine the inguinal region, the genitalia (if male) and perform a rectal examination.

The examiner will normally not require you to do either a genital or rectal examination, but volunteering that you would do both of these examinations normally shows the examiner that you recognise the importance of both in assessing abdominal pathology.

Station extension

A full abdominal examination including eyes, hands and regional lymph nodes will normally take longer than 5 minutes. Thus, in a 5-minute station, the instructions for the candidate will be quite specific e.g.:

E Palpate this patient's abdomen and tell me what you are doing at each stage.
or
E Look at this patient's abdomen and comment on what you can see.

Alternatively, a full abdominal examination does not normally take 10 minutes. Thus in both 5- and 10-minute stations, there is often an opportunity for extending the station to make it more challenging. In addition, those who are responsible for setting OSCEs are aware that all students will be expecting to examine an abdomen and will look to extend the station to discriminate very good from borderline students.

125

Typical extensions include:

- Single-contrast barium enema pictures showing complete large bowel obstruction
- The examiner may ask you to discuss:
  - the causes of hepatic/splenic enlargement
  - the use and site of stomas (Figures 10 & 12)
  - the psycho-social implications of stomas
  - the complications of gallstones
- An intravenous urogram
- A CT scan of an aortic aneurysm.

GASTROINTESTINAL

Suggestions for further practice

There are two distinct stages to developing competence in abdominal examination. Firstly, you must develop a technique which:

- is well practised and second nature
- is comprehensive and thorough
- is likely to detect pathological abnormalities.

This can be achieved by constant practice on patients/simulated patients/fellow students/housemates, etc. However, it is important that you do not develop bad habits and it is essential that you regularly expose your technique to a critical eye on a regular basis. Ward-based junior doctors are an ideal source for such a critical eye.

Once you have developed a competent technique for abdominal examination, you should actively seek out patients with abnormal abdominal signs.

- Liver abnormalities: oncology, hepatobiliary and haematology clinics and units
- Splenic abnormalities: haematology and oncology clinics
- Palpable kidneys are rare in general medical and surgical wards, but are common on renal and transplant units and clinics.
- Stomas and colonic masses: lower GI clinics and operating theatres.

126

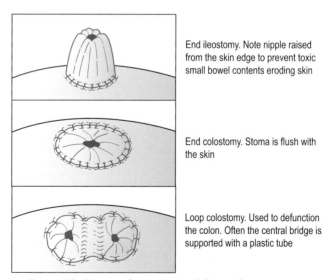

End ileostomy. Note nipple raised from the skin edge to prevent toxic small bowel contents eroding skin

End colostomy. Stoma is flush with the skin

Loop colostomy. Used to defunction the colon. Often the central bridge is supported with a plastic tube

Figure 12 Commonly occurring abdominal stoma types

Lymph nodes

Level:	**
Setting:	A patient or student volunteer
Time:	5 minutes

Task

E Show me how you would examine for lymphadenopathy in this patient.

S Would you like me to include or exclude the groins in this examination?

E No, you can leave the groins in this particular case.

Response

The examiner wants you to be able to demonstrate your knowledge of the sites of lymph node groups and your understanding of lymph node drainage. Once again basic surface anatomical knowledge is central to a good answer. The following lymph node groups should be examined in turn (Figure 13). Start with the patient sat up and examine the head and neck nodes from behind:

- sub-mental, sub-mandibular and occipital
- cervical
- supra-clavicular and infra-clavicular.

Start with the sub-mental nodes just under the chin, move your fingers to just below the angle of the mandible (sub-mandibular). Continue backwards to the pre- and post- auricular nodes. Now feel the cervical nodes, which run along the internal jugular vein, palpate for these along the anterior border of the sternocleidomastoid muscle. At the bottom of this muscle, move your hands backwards again to the supra-clavicular nodes. Finally try to remember the occipital nodes. (See Examination 6: Neck Examination.)

A good aide-memoir is that the shape of your examination is a 'Z' (think about how you are moving your hands along the jaw, down the neck and then to the supra-clavicular fossa).

Next, turn the patient towards you and examine the axillary lymph nodes as described in breast examination:

- Axillary

Examine the right axilla with your left hand and vice versa. Support the weight of the patient's arm with your other hand (practice on a friend to get used to your body position). (See Examination 9: Breast.)

127

EXAMINATION SKILLS

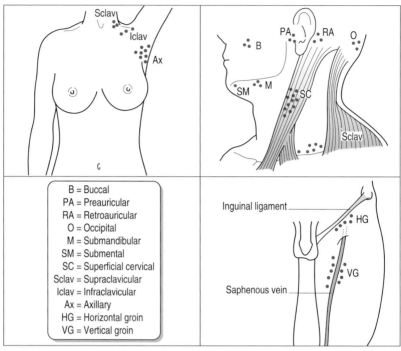

B = Buccal
PA = Preauricular
RA = Retroauricular
O = Occipital
M = Submandibular
SM = Submental
SC = Superficial cervical
Sclav = Supraclavicular
Iclav = Infraclavicular
Ax = Axillary
HG = Horizontal groin
VG = Vertical groin

Figure 13 Examining the lymphatic system. (a) Diagram of the palpable lymph nodes in the neck. In the neck, the patient should be examined from behind and each lymph node group examined in turn. (b) Diagram of the palpable lymph nodes of the upper limb and breast. In anatomical text books, the axillary nodes are separated into anterior, posterior, lateral, central and apical. When performing a cilinical examination it is very difficult to differentiate between these groups. (c) Diagram of the palpable lymph nodes in the groin and lower limb. These nodes are in two distinct groups. The vertical group follows the great saphenous vein at the saphenofemoral junction (2.5 cm below the inguinal ligament). Lymph then drains in to the horizontal group which lies just distal to the inguinal ligament

Finally lie the patient down.

- Epitrochlear
- Para-aortic
- Groin.

The para-aortic nodes are almost never palpable except in large lymphomas. Remember the aorta bifurcates just below the umbilicus.

Remember that whenever you feel a lymph node there are three further requirements of the examination:

1. The area draining to the involved node
2. Other lymph node groups
3. The liver and **spleen** (other components of the reticulo–endothelial system).

Areas draining to lymph node fields include:

- Inguinal: leg, abdominal wall below umbilicus (front and back), buttock, perineum (including scrotum and anal canal)
- Axilla: arm, chest wall and abdominal wall above the umbilicus (front and back), breast
- Cervical: head and neck, including the oral cavity, larynx and pharynx.

Remember that intra-abdominal malignancy can metastasise to the left supraclavicular nodes.

Comment

The examiner is likely to stop you at any time to enquire which nodes you are feeling for and which organs and tissues they drain. Have the answers ready.

Remember any time you feel a swelling: site, size, shape, surface, consistency, edges, fixation (superficial and deep), temperature, tenderness, overlying skin:

- **Size**: normal lymph nodes are usually less than 1 cm in diameter and ovoid. Nodes larger than 1 cm are more likely to be significant.
- **Consistency**: normal nodes are smooth and mobile. Hard nodes are typical of carcinoma, rubbery nodes of lymphoma; fluctuence is occasionally seen in tuberculosis. Pathological lymph nodes, particularly those involved in a malignant process often matt together, forming a nodular mass.
- **Tenderness**: seen in infection and some carcinomas.
- **Overlying skin**: tethering is seen in carcinomas; erythema and increased temperature suggest infection.
- **Fixation**: deep fixation is much more likely to be associated with a malignant than benign process.

Suggestions for further practice

Patients with lymphadenopathy are relatively uncommon. Lymph node examination is a routine part of the examination in surgical oncology. Haematology, medical oncology and HIV/AIDS clinics frequently have patients with generalised lymphadenopathy.

Station extensions

Because localised and generalised lymphadenopathy are often secondary to disease in a system outside the lymphatic system itself, diagnosing a patient with lymphadenopathy can be difficult. Because of this, station extensions tend to focus on the candidate's understanding of the potential underlying causes of lymphadenopathy and how you might investigate such a patient. Answering these questions in an organised way is a further example of appropriate usage of your 'surgical sieve'.

E What are the common causes of lymphadenopathy?

S Lymphadenopathy can be localised or generalised. The commonest causes of localised lymphadenopathy are local infection, metastatic disease and lymphoma whilst generalised lymphadenopathy is more likely to be due to systemic infection such as infectious mononucleosis or HIV/AIDS, lymphoma and some rare non-malignant diseases such as sarcoid or connective tissue disease.

E How would you investigate a patient with generalised lymphadenopathy?

S I would organise some blood tests including a blood count and differential white count and an ESR and CRP, particularly if I suspected an infective or inflammatory cause. Viral titres may be useful if glandular fever is suspected. I would arrange a chest X-ray to exclude pulmonary causes or mediastinal lymphadenopathy. If lymphoma is likely I would perform a CT scan of the chest and abdomen. If all other investigations were normal I would proceed to organising a lymph node biopsy.

Breast

Level:	*/**
Setting:	A patient or student volunteer with 'strap on' breasts or a real patient with a breast lump
Time:	5 minutes

Task

E   I want you to imagine that this lady is 55 years old and has come to see you complaining of a lump in her right breast. Show me how you would examine her.

Comment

Breast examination was always an examination rarity prior to the development of 'realistic' breast models. Today it is a common OSCE station, not only because it is a very important clinical examination, but also due to the availability of more lifelike, simulated breast models. There are two basic forms of breast models utilised in clinical skills settings. Figure 14a shows the older version, which is a simple latex model of the breast alone. Figure 14b shows the more recent 'strap-on' model, which permits examination of the axilla and appropriate patient positioning and interaction. The simple breast model is normally embedded with a simulated abnormality that feels like a physical breast lump and the abnormality serves as the stimulus for further questioning. In this case, the examiner will ask you to feel the breast rather than perform a breast examination.

For the purposes of this station, we will consider the 'strap-on' variety of breast simulator (Figure 14b) or a real patient with a breast lump.

Procedure

131

1. **Introduction:** Introduce yourself in a standard manner and acknowledge the patient's embarrassment if they look anxious. Request a chaperone.
2. **Inspection:** Ask the patient to remove clothing from above her umbilicus and sit with her legs up and together on the bed with her arms down by the side. Inspecting a patient from directly in front can be intimidating so inspect from the side of the bed, whilst standing adjacent to the patient's feet. Look for:

   * **Symmetry:** (most women are slightly asymmetrical. A variation of less than one bra cup size is considered normal)
   * **Skin changes:** inflammation, puckering, peau d'orange[5]

---

[5] French = 'orange skin'

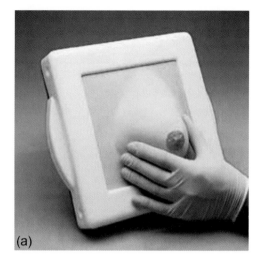

(a)

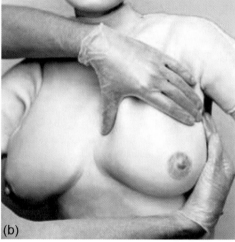

(b)

Figure 14(a) Traditional breast model; most frequently utilised to discuss clinical findings. **(b)** Modern 'strap-on' simulated breasts utilised to assess breast examination skills. Image courtesy of Limbs & Things

- **Nipple changes:** retraction, discharge, colour change
- **Obvious masses.**

Ask the patient to raise both arms above the head and look again for tethering and any masses.

3. **Palpation:** The patient's head should be raised at about 30° from the horizontal. This can be achieved with pillows or by folding the examination table. Start with the left breast. Ask the patient to raise the left arm behind her head. The breast should be palpated in six sections as illustrated in Figure 15. Until recently the custom was to palpate the breast with the flat

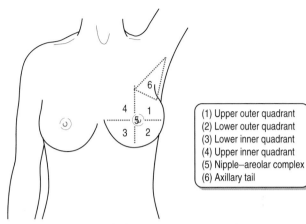

(1) Upper outer quadrant
(2) Lower outer quadrant
(3) Lower inner quadrant
(4) Upper inner quadrant
(5) Nipple–areolar complex
(6) Axillary tail

Figure 15 Breast examination. With the patient supine on the examining couch and with his/her arm behind his/her head, the six sectors are felt in turn

of the hand, much like abdominal palpation, more recently the trend is to use the tips of the fingers, as this is thought to be a more sensitive approach. Your hand should be placed flat on the skin and the distal interphalangeal joints should be gently flexed.

Next examine the axilla. This can be done again with the patient sat up. You must attempt to relax pectoralis major to get good access, so rest the patient's left forearm on your left forearm and briefly feel the lateral border of pectoralis major to make sure it is relaxed. Place the tips of the fingers of your right hand gently into the lower part of the axilla pressing the axillary tissue against the rib cage. Work up the axilla, palpating all the time until the tips of your fingers are high up in the apex. Repeat the process on the right but this time support the right forearm with your right arm and palpate with the fingers of the left hand.

4. **Maintain dignity:** The breast examination is intimate. Thank the patient and make sure that their breasts are covered before leaving or turning to the examiner.

133

Core skill	Breast examination

1. Introduce yourself, explain the procedure and request a chaperone
2. Position patient sat up on bed
3. Inspect slightly from the side with patient's hands by her side and then above her head
4. Palpate the six sectors
5. Palpate each axilla in turn
6. Cover breasts
7. Describe findings

Typical follow up questions

During the examination, the student finds a 2 cm lump in the upper outer quadrant of the right breast.

E How would you investigate this lump?

S I would perform triple assessment.

E What do you mean by triple assessment?

S Triple assessment refers to clinical examination, breast imaging and biopsy (not clinical examination, mammography and fine-needle aspiration!).

E What sort of imaging might be appropriate?

S Commonly this is mammography with or without ultrasound but it depends on the patient's age.

E Why does it depend on the patient's age?

S Mammography is only sufficiently sensitive in women over 35.

E What sort of biopsy may be appropriate?

S Fine-needle aspiration cytology is the commonest technique that I have seen, but I believe that wide-bore core cut biopsy is becoming more popular.

Comment

The student appears to have handled this station well. Breast disease is exceptionally common in both a hospital and community setting. Although the management of breast disease following diagnosis has become highly specialist over the last 10 years, it is very important that young doctors know how to recognise and diagnose breast problems. For specialists dealing with breast disease, pre-operative diagnosis is a central principle. Making an exact diagnosis without resorting to highly invasive tests allows the breast team to minimise distress and uncertainty to the patient. This is because the patient can be fully informed about their likely 'patient journey' and make informed choices about surgery, radiotherapy, chemotherapy and post-operative care before being subjected to invasive surgery. Triple assessment is the 'gold-standard' accepted method for making a pre-operative diagnosis. Most triple assessment in a modern hospital is performed during a single patient visit to outpatients and has very high diagnostic accuracy.

Station Extensions

In many ways the management of breast disease has led the way in developing a multidisciplinary approach to the management of serious illness. This multidisciplinary ethos is often reflected in examinations and you may be asked to comment on:

- the psycho-social aspects of a cancer diagnosis
- the psychological and sexual impact of mastectomy
- the possibility of breast reconstruction
- the value of breast screening.

Suggestions for further practice

Because the management of breast disease has become more specialist, many hospitals may have no breast service at all and refer their patients to another centre. It is possible that you will not be routinely allocated an experience of breast-disease management during your time at medical school. Nevertheless, nearly one in 10 women in the UK will develop breast cancer in their lifetimes and over 50% of the female population will be seen at a breast clinic before their 60th birthday, so there is plenty of opportunity for familiarising yourself with breast disease, but you may have to seek out the experience yourself. Most breast clinics are delighted to see students.

Groin

Level:	**
Setting:	A patient with a lump in the groin
Time:	5 minutes

Task

E This is Mr Stevens, who is 65 years old. He has a swelling in his groin. Would you examine his groin and tell me what you are doing as you are going along. He is wearing underclothes and you do not need to remove them.

Comment

Groin examination remains a common case in clinical examinations. For the purposes of OSCEs, the groin examination is often separated from testicular examination because it is easier to recruit 'real' patients if the groin is to be examined in isolation. In addition, there are many patients in the community with chronic groin abnormalities such as herniae. However, any surgeon will tell you that the groin and testicular examination are both part of a standard abdominal examination. Thus, despite the presence of a real patient, this OSCE station remains slightly artificial.

Having said this, remember that the vast majority of groin swellings are due to hernias. This station is a test of your ability to examine a swelling and in particular to examine a hernia. However it is worth having in mind a differential diagnosis. The best memory skeleton is probably based on anatomical structures in the region.

Direct and indirect inguinal hernias are **by far** the commonest in surgical OSCEs. It is important to establish that the patient has a hernia as quickly as possible. You can then demonstrate and explain to the examiner the

ANATOMICAL STRUCTURES AND COMMON GROIN LUMPS
Inguinal hernia
Inguinal lymph nodes
Swelling related to structures in the inguinal canal – hydrocele of the cord, lipoma of the cord
Vascular structures – aneurysm of femoral artery, saphena varix
Femoral hernia

ANATOMICAL STRUCTURES AND COMMON GROIN LUMPS—Cont'd

Masses in the right iliac fossa (i.e. the abdomen) are usually relatively easy to differentiate from inguinal swellings:

Appendix mass

Caecal carcinoma

Crohn's mass

Ovarian tumours

Iliac lymph nodes

Box 4.3 Common groin lumps

Direct inguinal hernia

Indirect inguinal hernia

Femoral hernia

Saphena varix

Lymph node

Ectopic testicle

Skin lump (sebaceous cyst/lipoma)

---

characteristics of hernias and the tests to differentiate between the different types going through the examination steps:

Inspection

Make sure the patient is lying flat with the groins exposed and ask the examiner if you should expose the external genitalia. Determine whether there is a

---

Core skill   Examining a lump in the groin

1. Introduce yourself to the patient
2. Request removal of all garments below umbilicus and ask the patient to stand up
3. Inspect
   - Scars, inflammation
   - Lumps, varicose veins
   - Ask patient to cough

GASTROINTESTINAL

4. Palpate
   - Locate lump and assess size, shape, consistency, etc.
   - With hand on lump ask patient to cough
   - Femoral pulse
   - Inguinal lymph nodes
5. Auscultate
   - Bowel sounds
   - Bruit

swelling at rest and, in particular, relate the swelling to the inguinal ligament; the most important anatomical landmark.

Now ask the patient to cough and look for a cough impulse. If there is a cough impulse, the patient has a hernia. Now look at the shape of the swelling:

- If it goes into the scrotum, it is almost certainly an indirect inguinal hernia.
- If it is sausage shaped along the line of the inguinal ligament, it is almost certainly an indirect inguinal hernia.
- If it has a more rounded shape and points directly to the ceiling, it is most likely to be a direct inguinal hernia.
- If the swelling is in the groin skin crease, it is likely to be a femoral hernia.

Therefore, at the end of inspection you may well have a very good idea of which type of hernia you are dealing with.

Palpation

First confirm that the swelling has a palpable cough impulse. Now feel for the anterior superior iliac spine and the pubic tubercle (you do need to practice feeling for this, but you can practice on yourself):

- If the swelling arises above this line, it is an inguinal hernia.
- If it arises below this line, it is a femoral hernia.

It is traditional for students to be expected to differentiate direct and indirect inguinal hernias. The deep inguinal ring is situated half way along the inguinal ligament. With the patient lying flat, reduce the hernia and press with one finger firmly over the deep ring. If the hernia can be controlled with this manoeuvre it is an indirect hernia.

Reduce the pressure a little over the deep ring and get the patient to cough. You can usually feel the hernia move under your finger and often see the swelling move along the inguinal canal. If the hernia is not controlled by pressure over the deep ring, the swelling will be seen medial to the deep ring on coughing and it is a direct hernia.

Many undergraduate textbooks emphasise the point about the relationship of the neck of the sac to the pubic tubercle. The student is told that if the neck of the hernia is below and lateral to the pubic tubercle it is a femoral hernia, and if the hernia is above and medial, it is an inguinal hernia. In reality it is much less complicated:

- If the hernia is above the inguinal ligament, it is an inguinal hernia.
- If the swelling goes into the scrotum, it is an inguinal hernia.
- If the swelling arises below the inguinal ligament, it is a femoral hernia.

Remember that sometimes a femoral hernia may not have a cough impulse. If the neck of the sac is very tight or occluded by, for example, a plug of omentum, the increase in intra-abdominal pressure on coughing may not be transmitted to the hernia.

Two further steps:

- Explain to the examiner that you would examine the testes.
- Having examined the patient lying down, if you have determined that it is a hernia and what type of hernia it is, it is not necessary to examine the patient standing up. If you have not elicited all the information, then repeat the examination with the patient standing.

Percussion
Not necessary unless there is a large irreducible swelling, when it may be helpful to determine whether there is bowel in the swelling.

Auscultation
Again not necessary unless again there is a large irreducible swelling whose nature is uncertain.

You may be asked to comment on two further aspects:

1. **Is the hernia strangulating/strangulated?** A surgical emergency. The hernia will be painful, and the overlying skin may be inflamed.
2. **Is the hernia reducible?** Tender irreducible hernias are a surgical urgency because of the risk of strangulation. Reducibility refers to reduction under mild/moderate pressure. Extreme pressure on a hernia may cause a strangulated hernia to fall back into the abdominal cavity and stay strangulated (a bit of a disaster if you think about it!). This is called *reductio en masse*.

Less common lumps in the groin

Saphena varix. A saphena varix is a dilatation at the top of the long saphenous vein due to valvular incompetence. It may reach the size of a walnut. They are soft and boggy and disappear completely when the patient is supine. They may, however, have a cough impulse. They also may demonstrate a fluid thrill.

Core skill	Examination of hernia

Inspection

1. Patient lying flat with groins exposed
2. Relate the swelling to inguinal ligament
3. A hernia is present if there is a cough impulse
4. Look at shape of swelling:
   - If in scrotum – probably an indirect inguinal hernia
   - If sausage shaped along inguinal ligament – then indirect inguinal hernia
   - If more rounded and points to ceiling – direct inguinal hernia
   - If in groin crease – probably femoral hernia

Palpation

1. Determine line between anterior superior iliac space and pubic tubercle
   - Above this line – inguinal
   - Below line – femoral
2. Reduce hernia and press with one finger over deep inguinal ring (halfway along inguinal ligament)
   - If this stops reappearance – indirect hernia

Skin lumps. Sebaceous cysts and large lipomata are not uncommon in this area and have the same characteristics as elsewhere.

Ectopic testis. Although rare, this is a perfect example of how groin examination cannot be taken in isolation. Very often, males with ectopic testes have an associated indirect inguinal hernia. The hernia may obscure the testis but scrotal examination will reveal an absent testis on the side of the hernia.

Inguinal lymphadenopathy. Superficial and deep inguinal nodes can become enlarged due to infection, inflammation, local malignancy or systemic disease. It is uncommon to find a solitary enlarged node in isolation.

Notes on orthopaedic examination

Nowhere does the general inspection on first contact give you more information than in examination of the patient with an orthopaedic problem. An impression of gait, posture, degree of discomfort and general health can be made within seconds of seeing a new patient. This skill is invaluable in orthopaedic examination to help focus your mind on the areas of the physical examination that are likely to be abnormal. Society and social etiquette today continually remind us that we must be slow to judge others on appearance, but adherence to this philosophy during a clinical examination can lead to oversights in diagnosis. Against social convention, you should become accustomed to looking for all non-verbal clues exhibited in the first few seconds of meeting your patient. A complete orthopaedic examination may take as long as 20 minutes. Thus, in most OSCE stations, you are asked to examine specific areas. The commonest areas are:

* hip
* knee
* back
* shoulder.

The principles of examination remain the same for each of these areas and follow the basic pattern:

* look
* feel
* move.

Look

When examining limbs it is essential that **BOTH** limbs are sufficiently exposed. Specifically look for:

* posture
* skin: scars, swellings, colour changes, dressings
* shape: is there wasting, length differences, bent bones?
* position: as well as posture, does the limb lie in a characteristic position (e.g. the shortening flexion and external rotation seen in fractured femoral neck)?

Feel

Look specifically for:

* skin warmth/cold, moist/dry
* lumps (treat as any lump)
* are there any palpable bony or joint deformities, steps or fluid
* any focal or diffuse tenderness.

Move

141

In principle it is always better to ask the patient to actively move a joint before asking them to relax and passively move the joint through its range of movement. This is done to ascertain how uncomfortable the action is and also to see if joint restriction is due to pain or physical prevention of movement. Active and passive movement assessment is a constant source of problems within an OSCE, because it depends on very specific instructions being given by the candidate to a patient who may not understand or comply the first time of asking. Your instructions need to be clear, simple and **WELL PRACTISED.** Try to use language that the patient is likely to understand immediately.

S   Please flex your hip joint.

Is likely to elicit a poorer response than:

S   Please move your thigh up towards my hand.

This is one part of the examination where your examiner will immediately recognise how often you have performed the examination on real people.

In contrast, if asked to present your findings, try to use the appropriate term for the specific movement that you are describing. Have a thorough grasp of the terms flexion, extension, abduction, adduction, medial and lateral rotation and circumduction.

Hip

Level:	*
Setting:	A patient or student volunteer
Time:	5 minutes

Task

E   Please examine this patient's right hip.

Comment

Almost invariably in OSCE examination stations, the patient will be lying supine on a couch, which determines the order in which you do things. You should start with the patient supine and ask them to stand and walk at the end of the examination.

Look

As mentioned in the introduction to this section, you should be assessing the patient from the moment you see them. You should observe how well they appear and ask yourself if they are lying comfortably on the examining couch.

Ideally, the patient should be exposed to the umbilicus with just the genitalia covered but this is often not practical in an OSCE, so the patient should be stripped to underwear. This means a minimum of clothing from the waist down. Most student volunteers are told to wear boxer shorts. Describe in detail what you can see remembering that hip examination is a **comparative** examination in which you are contrasting your findings with the contra-lateral limb. For example:

S   The right leg is lying in an externally rotated position when compared to the left.

An estimation of apparent comparative limb length can be made at this stage.

S   The right leg appears to be shorter than the left.

The presence of real or apparent limb shortening can be confirmed using a simple measuring test. A tape measure may be available at the station, but it is not a bad thing to get used to carrying one with you into exams. Apparent leg length = pelvic tilt + leg length, and is measured between the umbilicus and the medial malleolus. True leg length measurement eliminated the effect of pelvic tilting and is measured between the anterior superior iliac spine and the medial malleolus. Again this can appear clumsy unless it is sufficiently practised. Causes that shorten the leg are more common than those that lengthen it and include congenital growth deficiencies; infections

143

LOCOMOTOR

such as osteomyelitis, tumours, fractures, Perthes disease and slipped femoral epiphysis.

Feel

There is rarely much to feel when examining the hip in an adult. Pain may be apparent on deep palpation in the groin and gross swelling can sometimes be felt in a thin patient.

Core skill	Hip examination

A basic check list for examination of the hip is:

1. Comment on any:
   - swelling/skin discolouration
   - deformity
   - muscle wasting
   - scars
2. Comment on any tenderness over the joint (and allow for it in your examination)
3. Ask the patient to move the joint through: flexion, rotation, abduction, adduction and extension and estimate any restriction in movement
4. Passively move the joint through the same movement and look for differences compared to the active movements
5. Measure true leg length
6. Ask the patient to walk and observe the gait
7. Comment on any restriction or pain on movement

Move

The hip is a modified synovial ball and socket joint and consequently, has a wide range of movement. To complicate matters further, unless the pelvis is immobilised, the spine and pelvis will contribute to apparent hip movement.

Flexion

Ask the patient to bring their knee up towards their chest. Ask them to repeat the movement with your hand preventing the iliac crest from moving simultaneously. When the patient is at maximum flexion, hold the leg and ask the patient to relax and attempt to flex the hip further. At this point, you will be flexing the patient's hip passively, stabilising the iliac crest with your other hand and looking at the patient's face to make sure you are not causing excessive pain. **This is a complex procedure** and must be **practised** frequently if you want to look slick. Finally, you should test for a fixed flexion deformity using a Thomas[6] test. Basically, patients with a fixed flexion deformity of the hip can compensate for this by flexing the

---

[6] Hugh Owen Thomas (1834–1891) British Orthopaedic Surgeon, also Thomas splint

lumbar spine. Therefore such a deformity cannot always be seen with the patient lying supine. A Thomas test involves removing the lumbar lordosis by flexing the *unaffected* hip (placing your other hand underneath the patient to make sure that the lumbar lordosis is obliterated). If the patient has a fixed flexion deformity the affected leg will rise off the table.

Abduction and adduction

Once again before asking the patient to cross their legs, you must prevent movement of the pelvis by grasping the opposite iliac crest and laying the forearm across the pelvis. The patient is then asked to abduct and adduct each leg in turn. Following maximal active movement the leg is held and passive abduction assessed.

Rotation

This should be tested in several positions. Probably the most accurate method is with the patient prone and the knee flexed (see Figure 16). With the hips extended, the legs should be rolled on the couch using the feet as indicators. If possible the patient should be asked to roll over and the knees flexed to 90° and rotation can be assessed using the tibia as an indicator. Rotation can also be assessed with the patient supine with the hip flexed and seated. None of these techniques is 'wrong' but, as with all examination skills, whichever method you use make sure you have repeatedly practised it.

Extension

This is difficult to assess, but if you have positioned the patient prone to examine rotation, you can estimate extension at this time.

Examination of gait

It is possible that the examiner will not require you to examine the gait of the patient because of time limitations in a short OSCE station. However, you must indicate that you would do it as a matter of routine. If you are required to do so, then ask the patient politely to stand up straight. Observe for any

145

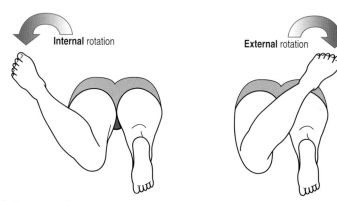

Internal rotation   **External** rotation

Figure 16 Examining hip rotation with the patient in a prone position: the hip should be able to rotate about 40° in either direction

scoliosis[7] (side-to-side/lateral curvature of the spine), lordosis[8] (accentuation of the lumbar curvature of the spine) or kyphosis[9] (posterior curvature of the thoracic spine) or any signs of pain when straightening. Ask the patient to walk a few steps and observe for an obvious limp and note the characteristics of the limp. Try to observe the overall appearance of the gait; does the patient swing their limbs, do they hobble? Describe **exactly** what you see. Many students worry unnecessarily about gait examination because there are many complex definitions and descriptions in the text books. The accurate and precise assessment of gait is a complex postgraduate skill that takes many years to acquire and you will not be expected to make diagnoses based on rare or subtle gaits, BUT there are several surgical diseases which are common and produce characteristic gaits, which may form part of an undergraduate OSCE station.

A note on Trendelenburg[10]

If the hip is painful, weak, dislocated or fractured, its stability is affected. As a result, the pelvis tilts down to the opposite side instead of tilting up when

Table 4.6 Common types of abnormal gait

Gait type	Description	Underlying cause
Antalgic (painful)	Patient leans towards painful hip and takes rapid heavy step followed by slow step on unaffected side	Osteoarthritis Trauma
Drunken	Patient walks with wide base, feet are raised excessively and placed carefully	Cerebellar pathology Alcohol intoxication
Festinating[11]	Short jerky steps becoming faster, but arms do not swing	Parkinson's disease
High stepping	Patient has foot drop so lifts leg up high to avoid scraping toe on the ground	Polio Multiple sclerosis
Trendelenberg	See Figure 17	Dislocation of the hip Fracture of the greater trochanter Slipped upper femoral epiphysis Polio Nerve root lesion

[11] Latin Festino = I hurry

[7] Greek skolios = crooked
[8] Greek lordos = bent backwards
[9] Greek kūphōsis = bent
[10] Friedrich Trendelenburg (1844–1924) German Surgeon

walking. This is because the muscles acting across the joint are not strong enough to stabilise the weight of the body through the hip joint. For some reason, students worry about this sign. Simply ask the patient to stand on one leg in order to test for hip stability (Figure 17). If the patient's body and pelvis sag to the side of the raised foot then the contra-lateral hip is weak and the test is positive.

Station extension

- You should be familiar with plain AP and lateral hip radiographs. You may be asked about the anatomical bony landmarks.
- You may be asked to comment on the surgical treatment of hip osteoarthritis, particularly hip replacement.

Suggestions for further practise

- Osteoarthritis is a very common, chronic disorder and there is a large resource for learning in the community and in primary care.
- Physiotherapists are experts at the diagnosis and treatment of chronic hip and knee disorders. Their anatomical knowledge is very good and physiotherapy clinics are frequently overlooked by undergraduates.

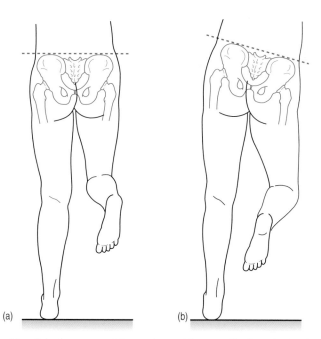

(a)   (b)

Figure 17 The Trendelenburg test: (a) a patient with normally functioning hip abductor muscles maintains a horizontal pelvis. (b) When the abductors are weak the pelvis tilts downwards on the more affected side

Knee

Level:	*/***
Setting:	A patient or student volunteer
Time:	5 minutes

E This patient is complaining of pain in his knees when walking. Would you examine the knees?

The anatomy of the knee joint, which we strongly recommend you revise prior to your OSCE, is complex and this makes knee examination quite difficult to master. However there are certain key anatomical features which will help you get a grasp of knee physiology and pathology (see Box 4.4). In addition, chronic soft-tissue knee pathology is extremely common and this is reflected in the frequency of knee examination stations in OSCEs. In common with all orthopaedic examinations you should:

- look
- feel
- move.

In addition, there are several 'special tests' in knee examination, which you should be familiar with. Some of these are more subtle and complex than others

Box 4.4	
Key points: Knee anatomy	
Joint type	The knee is a hinge joint articulating between the femoral and tibial condyles and the patella and patellar surface of the femur
Capsule	The capsule covers all articular surfaces and communicates with several of the surrounding bursae, particularly the suprapatellar and semimembranosus bursa
Capsular reinforcement	The capsule is reinforced and protected by the medial and lateral collateral ligaments on either side, the ligamentum patellae in front and the oblique ligament (an extension of the semimembranosus tendon) behind
Cruciate ligaments	Are named after their TIBIAL attachments and run obliquely across the joint. The anterior cruciate becomes taught when the knee extends and resists forward displacement of the tibia whilst the posterior cruciate becomes taught when the knee flexes and resists backward dislocation of the tibia

and probably beyond the scope of undergraduate learning. The more commonly used tests are discussed below to illustrate how tests have been specifically designed to recognise precise anatomical pathology.

Look

- Shape. Look for differences between the knees. Wasted quadriceps muscles markedly alter the knee's appearance. Sometimes gross bony or fluid (effusions and bursitis) swelling can be seen.
- Skin. Look for sinuses, bony growths and scars. Scars are very common even in younger people. The length and site of scars may give clues to underlying pathology. For example, a large lateral scar running vertically across the joint may indicate a previous knee replacement.
- Position at rest. Is there a valgus[12] (outward) or Varus[13] (inward) deformity. Is the knee partially flexed or hyperextended.

Feel

- Skin. Compare the temperature of each knee with the back of the hand. If you think that both knees are warm compare the warmth of the knees with an area of skin on the patient's thigh.
- Palpate the joint line. Bend the knee to about 45° and feel the medial joint line with the tips of your fingers. You should be able to feel the tibial tuberosity. Move your fingers from front to back asking the patient to tell you if he/she feels any discomfort. Similarly, feel the lateral joint line. Finally, place your fingertips deep in the popliteal fossa.
- Test for fluid. It is easy to look foolish when testing for an effusion if you are not well practised. There are two commonly used tests for fluid:

1. *The bulge test:* useful when only a little fluid is present. Massaging upwards on the medial side of the joint empties the medial compartment. Fluid is retained in the suprapatellar bursa by pressing just above the patella with the hand. The lateral side of the joint is then stroked down with the other hand whilst you observe for a bulge in the medial side of the joint.
2. *The patellar tap:* in this test, fluid in the suprapatellar bursa is emptied with your hand by massage. Fluid enters the joint and causes the patella to rise off the joint. A sharp push on the patella causes a 'tap' to be felt.

Move

- Flexion and extension. The knee is a modified hinge joint so it is capable of flexion and extension and at the end of extension it rotates slightly to allow 'locking'. *Quadriceps femoris* is the principal extensor muscle of the knee. It is supplied by the femoral nerve (L3,4). Flexion

149

---

[12] Valgus: Latin = knock-kneed
[13] Varus: Latin = bow-legged

is controlled through the tibial nerve (L5–S3) supplying the hamstring muscles. The biceps femoris passes lateral to the head of the fibula whilst semitendinosus and semimembranosus attach to the upper tibia. The patient should be asked to flex and extend the muscles themselves. The knee should be sufficiently flexible to allow the calf to meet the back of the thigh (about 160°).

- Medial and lateral collateral ligaments. With the joint held in extension, the ankle is tucked under one arm with both hands holding the knee and lower femur. The joint is then stressed by moving the tibia medially and laterally (varus and valgus) whilst the femur is fixed. The knee should not move AT ALL in this plane.
- Cruciate ligaments. This technique should be practised. The knee is flexed to 90° and the foot secured using your elbow. Using both hands, the upper end of the tibia is pulled forwards and backwards. If the tibia moves excessively anteriorly then the anterior ligament is lax whilst excessive posterior movements denote posterior ligament pathology.
- The McMurray[14] test. Hold the femur steady with the knee flexed. Using your other hand gently rotate the foot medially and laterally. If there is resistance to movement or pain then the test is positive and suggestive of meniscal injury.

Core skill   Knee examination

1. Show awareness to any discomfort for the patient
2. Expose and inspect both knees (thighs/calves)
3. Comment on any difference in temperature between the knees
4. Examine and comment on bony/synovial swelling
5. Examine for, and comment on, the presence of effusions
6. Demonstrate any differences in active and passive range of movements
7. Demonstrate any lateral and AP instability

150

Station extensions

Typically you may be asked:

E   What do you think may cause pain in the front of the knee?

S   Anterior knee pain is very common in athletes. Climbing stairs, squatting or kneeling, often exacerbates the pain. Anterior knee pain is also known as patella femoral syndrome and is believed to be due to an irritation on the under surface of the patella or knee cap, which can lead to softening and eventual loss of the cartilage lining the bone of the joint.

---

[14] Thomas Porter McMurray (1887–1949), British Orthopaedic Surgeon

Causes:
1. Misalignment: e.g. flat feet, knock knees, or internally rotated hips
2. Weak quadriceps muscles
3. Direct injury
4. Obesity.

E What would you expect to find in rheumatoid and osteoarthropathies?

S Patients with osteoarthritis are usually over 50 years and may be overweight. Pain is the principal symptom and is normally exacerbated by use, so it is often worse in the evening. After rest the patients often complain of stiffness. Swelling may occur and sometimes the patients may complain of the knee 'giving way' or locking. Normally, on examination the joint is not hot and there is rarely copious joint fluid.

Patients with rheumatoid arthritis of the knee tend to be younger and are more often female. In the early stages of the disease, the patient complains of pain and swelling and there is often a large effusion and the joint feels warm. As the disease progresses the joint erodes and movement may be reduced or lost.

E How might a meniscus injury present?

S Meniscal injuries or tears tend to occur when the knee is flexed and is over-rotated. These tears often occur in young adults during sports. Pain is instant and severe and sometimes the knee locks. Swelling appears within hours.

E What do you understand by the term 'locked' knee?

S A locked knee usually occurs at a particular point of flexion of the joint and indicates that the knee cannot be extended (i.e. straightened). It is associated with loose bodies in the joints interfering with its normal movement. The joint may' unlock' through the patient flexing and rotating the joint, causing the loose body to move out of the way. The commonest cause of a loose body is a meniscal tear.

151

Suggestions for further practice

- The knee is complicated. Read a 'classic' description of knee anatomy. Modern-day clinical skills units will have very detailed plastic models. Study them carefully. Pay particular attention to the ligaments and semilunar cartilages and the muscles responsible for knee stabilisation. Using the models, try to work out how the common types of injury occur.

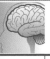

Ear, nose and throat (deafness)

Level:	**
Setting:	A patient with hearing loss
Time:	10 minutes

E Mr Jones is 60. He is complaining that he has a ringing in his ears and his wife says that he sometimes can't hear a thing. Show me how you would assess his hearing.

Comment

Otolaryngology is often under-represented in the curriculum of many undergraduate medical programmes given the enormous scale of problems affecting this system, particularly the ear. The reasons for the under-representation are numerous, but include:

- many ENT problems are managed in the community and many curricula focus on hospital-based care
- many ENT problems cause chronic mild-to-moderate disability and many patients self-manage
- many ENT problems are assessed and managed by non-medical practitioners who do not routinely teach medical students
- ENT surgeons tend to see the most severe cases only.

The lack of formal ENT learning opportunities in your programme is often not reflected in OSCEs. This is because there are many patients with chronic ENT conditions and there are some very good models. You must make sure that you are prepared for ENT OSCE stations by taking the initiative and gaining sufficient practice at ENT examination and exposure to patients with ENT conditions.

The examiner is attempting to establish the following:

- Can the candidate reliably assess deafness?
- Can the candidate differentiate between sensorineural and conduction deafness?
- Is the candidate aware of the potential causes of deafness?

Core skill	Examination of hearing loss
Talk in a normal voice to the patient	An informal assessment of the degree of hearing loss can be made based on how loud you need to speak. If there is no obvious difficulty in hearing then ask the patient if they can hear your watch ticking. Test each ear separately
Inspect	Are the auricular and periauricular tissues normal?
Otoscopy*	External auditory canal look for: • cerumen (wax) • foreign bodies • skin abnormalities • infection • eczema • tumour Tympanic membrane: • colour • mobility • surface anatomy
Weber's test and Rinne's test	To differentiate between sensorineural and conduction deafness.

*It is worth explaining to the examiner what you are looking for during otoscopy because the examiner cannot see exactly what you are doing.

Core skill	Using an otoscope

1. Choose a speculum which has a slightly smaller diameter than the external meatus
2. Pull the pinna gently backwards and upwards in adults or backwards and downwards in infants (this straightens out the auditory meatus)
3. Gently insert the tip of the otoscope into the external meatus whilst looking where you are going
4. Inspect the external canal
5. Inspect all parts of the tympanic membrane by gently varying the angle of the speculum
6. Withdraw the otoscope gently

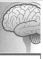

NEUROLOGICAL

Weber's test[15]

This test is performed by softly striking a 512-Hz (c one octave above middle c) tuning fork and placing it midline on the patient's forehead. If the hearing loss is conductive, the sound will be heard best in the affected ear. If the loss is sensorineural, the sound will be heard best in the normal ear. The sound remains midline in patients with normal hearing.

Rinne's test[16]

This test compares air conduction with bone conduction. The tuning fork is placed on the mastoid process. When the patient no longer can hear the sound, the tuning fork is placed adjacent to the external auditory meatus. In the presence of normal hearing or sensorineural hearing loss, air conduction is better than bone conduction. Therefore, sound is still heard when the tuning fork is placed adjacent to the ear canal. In the presence of conductive hearing loss, bone conduction is better than air conduction, and the sound is not heard when the tuning fork is placed adjacent to the canal.

Interpretation of these tests is shown in Table 4.7 (for deafness affecting the left ear).

Station extensions

E What further investigations might you consider performing to establish the cause and severity of this patient's deafness?

- **Pure tone audiometry.** This is used to determine hearing sensitivity. A series of pure tone thresholds are measured and plotted to produce an audiogram.
- **Tympanometry.** The pressure in the external auditory meatus is altered and at each setting, passing sound to the ear and measuring the sound energy reflected. A three-channel tympanometer is used – with separate channels for each function. This is a method to assess middle-ear compliance or to assess nerve deafness and glue ear in children.

Table 4.7 Interpreting Rinne's and Weber's tests

	Rinne's test	Weber's test
Sensorineural deafness Left ear	Air conduction > bone conduction (both diminished)	To opposite side (right)
Conduction deafness Left ear	Bone conduction > air conduction	To same side (left)

---

[15] Ernst Heinrich Weber (1795–1870) German physiologist not to be confused with Frederick Parkes Weber (1863–1962) (Sturge-Weber and Osler-Weber-Rendu syndromes) English physician
[16] Friedrich Heinrich Adolf Rinne (1819–1868) German ear-nose-throat surgeon

- **Electric response audiometry.** This is a type of electrophysiological hearing assessment in which electrodes are placed on the head, which emit frequencies that block out interference from background electrical activity such as normal brainwaves. The effect of pure sounds can then be assessed on different parts of the brain. Cochlear, brainstem and cortical responses to sound can be measured depending on the technique employed.
- **Acoustic reflexes.** These tests measure the changes in the ear's ability to conduct sound to the cochlea. It is often performed at the same time as tympanometry. The stapedius muscle is stimulated with sound waves and its degree of stapedius contraction is measured.

E   What are the different types of deafness and what are the more common causes?

Suggestions for further practice

We suggest that as a minimum you prepare by:
- attending a children's ENT clinic
- attending an adult's ENT clinic
- attending an audiometry clinic

Practice ear and mouth examinations on models in your skills lab, and as many patients as you can.

Table 4.8 Common causes of deafness

Type	Causes
Conduction deafness	
	Outer ear:
	• wax
	• foreign body
	Inner ear:
	• otitis media
	• cholesteatoma
	• otosclerosis
	• ruptured tympanum
Sensorineural deafness	Disorders of the cochlea:
	• congenital
	• infection
	• drugs (particularly aminoglycosides)
	• presbycusis (age-related deafness)
	• noise induced
	• Ménière's disease[17]

[17]   Prosper Ménière (1799–1862) French physician

Ear, nose and throat (oral cavity)

NEUROLOGICAL

Level:	**
Setting:	A head and neck mannequin
Time:	5 minutes

Task

E This patient (pointing to the mannequin) is complaining of a swelling inside his mouth. Show me how you would examine the oral cavity.

Comment

The oral cavity is another area of the body that often receives little attention in the undergraduate curriculum. It is frequently considered by students and their teachers to be the realm of dentists or oral surgeons. Most oral pathology is infective, traumatic or reactive, but oral malignancies are not uncommon and frequently present late because of the 'hidden' nature of the oral cavity. In addition, the development of realistic and robust head and neck mannequins means that oral and ENT examinations are becoming more common in OSCEs.

Inspection is the principal focus of examination of the oral cavity and it is easy to rush this aspect and miss important pathology. Because of this, we suggest that you inspect the mouth by taking each anatomical site in turn starting with the lips. A good light source is also essential, preferably using a fixed or head-mounted light.

The lips

Examine the lips both visually and by palpation. The vermilion border should be smooth, soft and pliable. Inflammation of the lips is called cheilitis and often manifests as 'chapping' or cracking. Cracking of the corner of the mouth (angular cheilitis) can be due to the following:

- localized infection (normally *Candida*)
- vitamin B and other nutritional deficiency
- overclosure of the jaws due to loss of normal dentition.

Oral mucous membranes

Be careful when describing oral mucosa as abnormal in colour or thickness. There is a great deal of natural physiological variation in colour and keratinisation. Evert the lips and look at the labial oral mucosa. This should be smooth, soft and well lubricated. Superficial aphthous ulcers and blocked salivary ducts (resulting in a mucocele) are common in this area. Next examine the buccal mucosa by asking the patient to open his/her mouth and gently press the buccal mucosa with a tongue depressor. Look for raised plaques and other abnormal lesions. The opening of the parotid duct can be seen just above the maxillary first molar tooth. Often saliva can be seen bubbling out of the duct. The saliva should be watery and clear.

Tongue

Ask the patient to protrude the tongue and try to touch the tip of his/her nose. This exposes the dorsal surface of the tongue.

Look for the taste buds:

- filiform papillae: numerous hair-like protrusions scattered uniformly across the dorsum of the tongue
- fungiform papillae: mushroom-like buds, less in number than the filiform papillae, but larger
- circumvallate papillae: 8–12 in number arranged uniformly in a delta shape at the junction of the anterior two-thirds and posterior third of the tongue.

The lateral border of the tongue can be visualised by gently grasping the tongue with a gauze swab and rotating it from side to side. The ventral aspect of the tongue is best visualised by asking the patient to place the tongue on the roof of their mouth with the mouth open. Look for the orifices of the submandibular ducts lying either side of the lingual frenulum. The ventral and lateral surfaces of the tongue are common sites of oral squamous carcinoma and the presence of masses in these areas should be carefully noted.

Palate

The hard palate is best visualised by an intraoral mirror. It is frequently more keratinised than the rest of the oral mucosa and this causes it to be a paler colour. It is also ridged. The soft palate can be visualised by depressing the tongue and asking the patient to say 'Ah'. The soft palate is usually pink. Deviation of the palate to one side may indicate neurological disease.

157

Tonsils

The tonsils form part of a collection of lymphoid tissue that surrounds the entrance to the GI and respiratory tracts. Waldeyer's[18] ring consists of the palatine tonsils, the lingual tonsil, the adenoids and other small collections of lymphoid tissue. The tonsillar pillars can be visualised by moving the tongue to one side using the tongue depressor. The tonsillar crypts often have food debris within them but when clean are very pink due to their vigorous blood supply.

Teeth and gums

A general inspection of the teeth and gums is essential for a thorough examination of the oral cavity. Changes in the gingiva can indicate both local and systemic

[18] Heinrich Wilhelm Gottfried von Waldeyer-Hartz (1836–1921) German Professor of Anatomy and Physiology

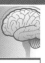

NEUROLOGICAL

disease. Tooth decay is often accompanied by gingival inflammation and retraction whilst they can be the first affected site of lichen planus, HIV or pemphigus. Extra and missing teeth can be a sign of inherited disorders such as Gardner's syndrome.

Core skill	**Examination of the oral cavity**

1. Introduce yourself, explain what you are going to do
2. Put on gloves and ensure a gauze swab, tongue depressor and a dental or laryngeal mirror is available. If they are not then ask
3. Adjust the light source so it is shining directly into the patient's mouth
4. Inspect (external).
   - facial or oral asymmetry
   - skin lesions
   - signs of 'syndromic' conditions, such as micrognathia
5. Inspect and palpate the lips: the vermillion should be smooth and soft
6. Open the mouth and depress the tongue to inspect. Make sure the light source is illuminating the area of inspection
7. Ask the patient to extend the tongue and examine the hard and soft palate and the uvula. If a dental mirror is available, carefully insert the mirror and look behind the teeth and the posterior aspect of the lips
8. Use a gauze pad to grip the edge of the tongue and extend it as far as possible. Ask the patient to raise their tongue, and view the ventral surface and the floor of the mouth
9. With a gloved hand, palpate the roots of the teeth, the gingiva and the vestibules, and with two hands (one inside the mouth and one outside) gently compress the walls and floor of the mouth
10. Examine the neck for lymph nodes (see station Examination 8)
11. Smell the patient's breath for evidence of infection, alcohol and tobacco use

Extension to station

The examiner is likely to ask you to describe the aetiology of oral cancer.

Smoking (both tobacco and marijuana), chewing tobacco and alcohol use have all been shown to increase risk of oral malignancy. Leukoplakia (white spots or patches around the oral cavity) can also be considered to be a risk factor, as over one-third of patients with leukoplakia will develop cancer if left untreated. Most commonly, oral cavity cancer is a squamous carcinoma.

Suggestions for further practice

- Make oral examination a routine part of your general clerking examination.
- Maxillo-facial and general dental practices are an underused resource and they are a great place to learn mouth examination

Interpretation skills

Introduction

In the early days of OSCE examinations, interpretation stations were often used to fill up space between a limited number of clinical skills stations. Interpretation stations are relatively easy for examiners to set and administer because:

- there is plenty of resource: radiographs, blood results, urine results, etc.
- they do not require patients or simulated patients
- they do not require specialised pieces of equipment
- in some cases, they are marked following the completion of the OSCE.

As OSCEs, OSCE setters and OSCE stations have become more sophisticated, interpretation stations have become a highly specialised method of assessing student competencies that are difficult to reliably assess in other ways.

Most interpretation stations follow a similar format:

1. You are presented with a small amount of information
2. You are asked to assimilate the information under the examination pressure
3. You are asked to comment on the information
4. You are given further information
5. You are asked to use the further information to expand upon your initial assumptions.

Some of the stations will have an examiner who will ask you questions and guide you. In others there will be no examiner and you will be asked to complete a written answer or, more recently, a computer-based answer.

Some stations may require you to complete a document such as a prescription sheet, referral letter or death certificate, which mimics those formal documents which you would find in your normal clinical life.

Interpretation stations are difficult to revise for, specifically because the potential source of data can be from any area of clinical medicine, but there are techniques that can improve your overall approach to these stations.

Endoscopic image

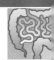

Level:	***
Setting:	Structured oral with examiner
Time:	5 minutes

Comment

Surgery is a practical discipline and surgeons, like many other doctors, have learnt to use their vision, smell, touch and hearing to maximise their diagnostic ability. The advent of endoscopy, high-definition video and modern imaging techniques like MRI scans has been embraced in the surgical world and many surgical OSCE stations will reflect this. Endoscopy is now an ESSENTIAL tool of the GI surgeon and images from endoscopies are often present in surgical patient's notes and the focus of multi-disciplinary team meetings. It is not surprising that endoscopic images are now a common part of interpretation stations in OSCEs.

Task

A 52-year-old has attended the endoscopy unit for investigations of abdominal pain.

The endoscopic image (Figure 18) was taken during the procedure.

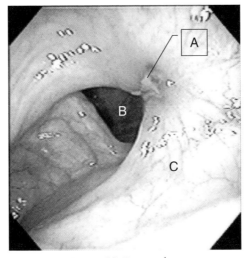

Figure 18 Peptic ulcer

161

GASTROINTESTINAL

E   What abnormality is shown and what is your diagnosis?

Response

The picture shows the terminal ileum. There is ulceration of the mucosa of the terminal ileum, which can be seen as a white eroded area (A). The mucosa shows oedema and erythema. The macroscopic appearances do not allow you to make a histological diagnosis, but Crohn's disease is the commonest cause of such an ulcer at the ileocaecal junction.

The diagnosis is made from the distribution of the ulceration. Ulcerative colitis only involves the colonic mucosa and whilst ulcerative colitis can be associated with backwash ileitis, it is not associated with ileal ulceration. Ulceration of the ileal and colonic mucosa can be associated with infectious enteritis, but in the UK, this would be rare.

E   What symptoms would you expect the patient to have?

Response

The expected symptoms would be colicky abdominal pain, exacerbated by eating. The patient may have symptoms related to an intra-abdominal abscess or fistula, such as swinging pyrexia. In addition, the patient may have general malaise, weight loss and symptoms from extra-intestinal manifestations of Crohn's disease such as:

- erythema nodosum
- aphthous mouth ulcers
- pyoderma gangrenosum
- conjunctivitis, iritis, uveitis
- arthropathy

Crohn's disease can affect the small bowel, the large bowel or both. Symptoms from small-bowel disease result from the thickened small bowel wall causing narrowing of the lumen. The pattern of the pain is small bowel colic, in which the small bowel is contracting hard to squeeze the small bowel contents through the narrowed lumen.

A fistula to the bladder may cause pneumaturia, whilst a fistula from the small bowel to the colon may result in diarrhoea, as parts of small intestine and colon are bypassed. An abscess would cause abdominal pain and fever.

Ulceration in the colon would cause the typical features of colitis. The more distal the colitis, the more the likelihood of visible blood in the stool.

E   What would biopsies of the small bowel show?

Response

The histology would show ulceration of the mucosa, with inflammation extending deep to the mucosa. It may also show granulomas.

You cannot say that inflammation would extend through the full thickness of the bowel wall, as a biopsy would only contain mucosa and sub-mucosa.

E How might you treat this patient?

Response

Medical treatment might include

- oral steroid therapy
- oral or rectal 5-aminosalicylic acid
- in severe cases, immunosuppressants such as azothiaprine

Surgery is considered when there is a failure of medical therapy or if there are complications, such as fistula or abscess. Given the relapsing nature of the condition, surgery is limited to what is necessary to manage the current problem.

The patient with Crohn's disease also requires continuous emotional support for this chronic, complicated illness; this support is necessary not only during acute attacks, but also during periods of remission.

Suggestions for further practice

Numerous atlases of endoscopic photographs are available in medical libraries. It is wise to familiarise yourself with the appearances of the areas, which are commonly visualised:

- stomach
- first part of duodenum
- common bile duct and ampulla of Vater (ERCP)
- colon
- terminal ileum.

Understanding how endoscopy is performed helps you orientate still photographs, so, once again, there is no substitute for hands-on experience. You should attend as many gastroscopy and colonoscopy lists as you can during your training.

Raised serum amylase

Level:	***
Setting:	Structured oral with examiner
Time:	10 minutes

Task

E A 35-year-old woman has been admitted to hospital with a 24-hour history of abdominal pain and vomiting and you are the admitting foundation trainee. Blood tests on admission show a serum amylase of 1936 IU/L (normal 10–87 IU/L). What other blood tests should be performed and why?

Comment

A very elevated serum amylase level (above four times the normal level) has very high sensitivity and specificity for acute pancreatitis, whilst moderate increases can be due to other causes such as:

- infection, e.g. mumps
- neoplasm, e.g. pancreatic carcinoma
- vascular, e.g. mesenteric ischaemia
- inflammatory, e.g. hepatitis, post-ERCP, peritonitis
- trauma, e.g. burns, posterior perforating duodenal ulcer, intestinal obstruction or perforation
- drugs, e.g. morphine and other opiates
- metabolic, e.g. renal failure, renal transplant, diabetic ketoacidosis.

Response

Acute pancreatitis is a very common acute medical problem. It is an important disease because it still has a mortality rate of around 10% and can be a fatal disease even for young patients.

Blood tests in acute pancreatitis are performed to:

- assess the severity of the disease and predict prognosis
- determine the initial management
- monitor the progress of the disease.

Assessing disease severity

Acute pancreatitis can be classified into mild and severe and several types of scoring system can be used to assess the severity of the attack. Perhaps the most widely used is the Ranson and Imrie scoring system (see Box 5.1). The presence

> **Box 5.1 Ranson and Imrie (Glasgow) criteria for assessing the severity of acute pancreatitis**
>
> 1. Age > 55 years
> 2. Hyperglycaemia in the absence of diabetes (glucose > 10 mmol/l)
> 3. Raised white cell count > 15×10^9/l
> 4. Raised urea > 16 mmol/l
> 5. Low PO_2 < 8 kPa
> 6. A low serum calcium < 2.0 mmol/l
> 7. A low albumen < 32 g/l
> 8. A raised lactate dehydrogenase > 600 IU/l
> 9. Raised liver transaminases (AST > 100 IU/l)

of three or more of these severity markers indicates a poor prognosis. You do not need to know in detail how to calculate the severity score, but you need to know that it is derived from a number of indicators.

Determining initial management and monitoring progress

The volume status of the patient can be assessed using the full blood count (high haemoglobin), haematocrit, urea, creatinine and sodium (hypernatraemia indicates relative water depletion). Patients with pancreatitis release many vasoactive peptides and enzymes locally into the abdominal cavity and into the circulation. Large volumes of fluid are sequestered into the abdomen and smaller quantities into the lung because of increased capillary permeability. This results in severe hypovolaemia and in severe cases, shock and circulatory collapse. Patients may lose up to 6 l of fluid in a very short space of time. The severity of these haematological and biochemical changes in combination with pulse, blood pressure and urine output will determine the requirements for fluid replacement. Repeating these tests during the course of the illness will allow fluid management to be titrated against clinical need.

A high white blood count and positive blood cultures may indicate systemic inflammation or infection. The routine use of antibiotics in severe pancreatitis is still subject to debate.

Measurement of blood gases is also useful as severe pancreatitis is associated with hypoxia and metabolic acidosis.

E   The patient has been treated with intravenous rehydration and is now stable. You have arranged an ultrasound examination of the abdomen, and the hand-written report states the following:

GASTROINTESTINAL

> ### Box 5.2 X-RAY Department University Hospital of St Elsewhere
>
> Liver, spleen and kidneys normal. Gaseous distension of the small bowel. Fluid collection around the pancreas with oedema of the body of the pancreas. Slightly distended gallbladder containing multiple small gallstones. The common bile duct is 5 mm in diameter.

How do you interpret the results and how should the patient be managed?

Response

The findings are typical of acute pancreatitis. The vast majority of patients (90%) have oedema of the pancreas rather than pancreatic necrosis, which is associated with severe pancreatitis. Magnetic resonance imaging cholangiopancreatography (MRCP) is becoming more widely used in pancreatic disease. Although not as sensitive as ERCP, MRCP is safer, non-invasive and fast, and it provides images useful in guiding clinical decisions. Pancreatic necrosis is best seen on contrast-enhanced CT scan.

The two major causes of acute pancreatitis are alcohol abuse and gallstones. The presence of the latter on the scan report indicates that these are the likely precipitating factor. The common bile duct is upto 5 mm in diameter up to age 50 and the upper limit of normal then increases by 1 mm per decade (e.g. 9 mm at age 90).

Patients with mild gallstone-induced pancreatitis are managed conservatively with rest, intravenous fluids, analgesia, oxygen and naso-gastric aspiration.

When resolved, the patient should be advised to undergo laparoscopic cholecystectomy. Ideally this should be within 1 month of discharge to reduce the chances of a further attack of pancreatitis.

Station extensions

Potential extensions are numerous and may focus on the aetiology of pancreatitis or its physical and psychosocial impact. A typical example may be:

E Tell me about other causes of acute pancreatitis?

Suggestions for further practice

Acute pancreatitis is a common cause of emergency admission. Many patients are admitted outside normal working hours, so you are more likely to see such patients whilst on call.

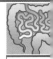

Table 5.1 Common causes of acute pancreatitis

1. Biliary disease (40%)	Caused by a gallstone passing down the common bile duct and lodging in the sphincter of Oddi[1]
2. Alcohol (35%)	Can occur in anyone taking excessive alcohol. Normally in patients who have been drinking heavily for 5–15 years but can occur in occasional drinkers following a binge
3. Post-ERCP (4%)	The risk is increased if the endoscopist is inexperienced. The exact cause is unknown
4. Trauma	Pancreatic injury occurs more often in penetrating injuries (e.g., from knives, bullets) than in blunt abdominal trauma (e.g. road traffic accidents)
5. Drugs	Many drugs can cause pancreatitis including azothiaprine, oestrogens, tetracycline, methyldopa and chemotherapy
6. Infection	Several infectious diseases may cause pancreatitis, especially in children. These cases of acute pancreatitis tend to be milder when compared to biliary or alcohol-induced pancreatitis. Viral causes include mumps, Epstein—Barr and coxsackie, whilst bacterial causes include *Mycoplasma pneumoniae, Salmonella* and *Campylobacter*

[1] Ruggero Oddi (1864–1913) Italian anatomist and surgeon

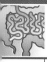

Chest radiograph

GASTROINTESTINAL

Level:	***
Setting:	Structured oral with examiner
Time:	10 minutes

Task

E A 45-year-old man has been admitted with abdominal pain, anorexia and weight loss to your ward. He is a heavy smoker and drinker. On examination he looks cachexic, he has a temperature of 38.4°C and he appears in pain. He is not very co-operative, which makes abdominal examination difficult, but he is diffusely tender and his abdomen is rigid. How would you proceed?

Response

This station is set not just to test your ability to interpret a chest X-ray, but also to assess your handling of a patient suffering several chronic underlying pathological processes. It is set as an interpretation station because of the difficulty in getting such a patient for an OSCE. The station can be made as hard or as easy as the examination setters' desire. Consequently, it is difficult to practice specifically for this type of station.

The important features here are the abdominal pain and temperature. The smoking history and pyrexia raise the possibility of a respiratory problem such as pneumonia. Tell the examiner that you know that respiratory problems can sometimes present with upper abdominal pain and vice versa. The heavy alcohol intake may indicate a liver problem and the abdominal pain obviously suggests acute intra-abdominal pathology.

The fact that the patient is unco-operative makes you more reliant on the result of investigations, but every attempt should be made to carry out a thorough history and examination, and talking to relatives or friends if they are available.

The investigations you could justify on admission are:

- full blood count – haemoglobin, haematocrit, raised white cell count, macrocytosis secondary to alcohol
- liver function tests – alcohol consumption
- urea and electrolytes – evidence of salt and water depletion, renal failure
- blood cultures – pyrexia
- blood gases
- blood sugar
- supine abdominal and erect chest radiograph.

E I would like you to look at this chest radiograph (Figure 19) and tell me what you think.

GASTROINTESTINAL

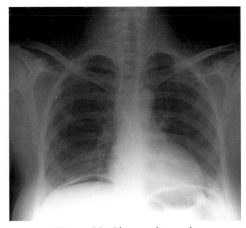

Figure 19 Chest radiograph

Comment

Chest radiograph interpretation is an important core skill and they are very common in OSCEs, appearing as part of a 5 or 10 minute station.

It may show abnormalities in the:

- lung/airway
- heart and mediastinum
- soft tissue
- skeleton
- sub-diaphragmatic.

Core skill Interpretation of a chest radiograph

1. Check the name, date and orientation of the film
2. State if it is an AP film (marked as such – causes apparent cardiomegaly)
3. Describe any obvious abnormality in the lung fields or heart shape:
   - Use upper, mid and lower zone to describe site of any problem
   - Need lateral film to localise to lobes (because of the direction of the fissures)
4. If there are no abnormalities (and at the end) check and comment on:
   - Any problems behind the heart (as long as good penetration)
   - Any bulkiness of the hila (lymph nodes, tumour, vascular – pulmonary hypertension)
   - Retrosternal goitre
   - Presence of both breast shadows in a female patient
   - Skeleton (ribs, humerus, clavicle)
   - Soft tissues

169

Continued

| Core skill | Interpretation of a chest radiograph—Cont'd |

5. Lungs:
   - Upper lobe collapse causes tracheal deviation
   - Lower lobe collapse causes mediastinal shift and the left lobe collapses as a triangle behind the heart
6. The middle lobe collapses as a triangle adjacent to the right heart with loss of the border

In the film for this station, the important abnormality is the presence of free gas underneath the diaphragm. It is frequently seen on the right side only because free gas on the left is often obscured by gas in the fundus of the stomach, but in this case is clearly visible on both sides. The radiograph chosen for this station should have a significant amount of free gas (i.e. be obvious). In other words, once you have thought about free gas it should be fairly easy to recognise (as is the case in clinical practice).

Station extensions

The examiner may ask you about the indications for chest radiographs in surgery. Elective chest X-rays used to be mandatory for all patients undergoing elective surgery. This is now not the case because it has been shown that they have little benefit in reducing morbidity and mortality. The exceptions are:

- smokers (one packet per day for 20 years)
- ASA status >3
- acute and chronic cardiovascular disease
- acute and chronic respiratory disease
- chest radiation therapy in the preceding 6 months
- severe disability and/or difficulty in collecting medical history.

Suggestions for further practice

Chest radiographs are exceptionally common in clinical practice and the experts at assessing such images are radiologists. Find one who is willing to allow you to attend a reporting session and ask them to explain their system for reporting.

Abdominal radiograph

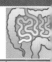

Level:	**
Setting:	Structured oral with examiner
Time:	5 minutes

E A 76-year-old woman is seen in the Accident and Emergency (A&E) Department with a 3-day history of abdominal pain, vomiting and constipation. The A&E doctor had arranged a plain abdominal radiograph. What does the radiograph show?

Response

In this situation you have not been given any information about the examination so the examiner expects you to be able to work out some aspects of the diagnosis from the history and radiograph. You would not be expected to determine all aspects of the case from the limited information you have been given.

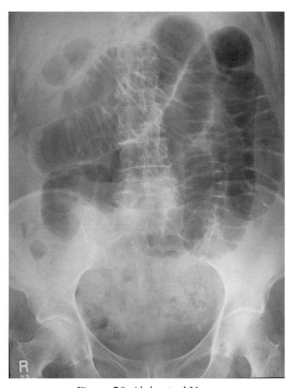

Figure 20 Abdominal X-ray

The radiograph shows distension of the small bowel with no large bowel distension. This can be discerned by the central location of the distended loops of bowel and the observation of the valvulae conniventes, which traverse the whole width of the small bowel (unlike the haustrations of the large bowel, which only traverse the width of the large bowel to a varying degree). It is very rare to have erect abdominal X-rays unless they are specifically ordered, so it is unusual to see fluid levels in the distended bowel.

Core skill   **Interpretation of an abdominal radiograph**

1. Check the name, date and orientation of the film
2. Describe any obvious abnormality in the distribution of gas in the abdomen:
   a. Small bowel dilatation
   b. Large bowel dilatation
   c. Oedema in the wall of the bowel
   d. Gas in the biliary tree
3. Look at the soft-tissue shadows:
   e. Psoas shadows
   f. Renal outline
   g. Along the line of the ureters for opacities
   h. Aortic or iliac calcification
4. Finally look at bony structures
   i. Scoliosis
   j. Osteoarthritis
   k. Spina bifida
   l. Lytic or sclerotic metastases

E On the basis of your interpretation of the radiograph, what would you look for on abdominal examination?

S The three commonest causes of small-bowel obstruction are hernia (inguinal, femoral, incisional, para-umbilical), adhesions and malignancy. Apart from looking for the cause of the obstruction; examining the hernial orifices, scars from previous abdominal surgery and signs of malignancy, such as abdominal masses, I would also look for the degree of abdominal distension and tenderness. A very distended, tender abdomen may indicate imminent bowel rupture. I would expect to hear high-pitched (obstructed) bowel sounds on auscultation.

E Having established a diagnosis of small-bowel obstruction secondary to a femoral hernia, what treatment is required before the patient is taken to the operating theatre for definitive management?

Comment

The examiner is telling you what the final diagnosis is and what the final treatment is, and wants you to fill in the gap about what should happen between diagnosis and definitive treatment. Treatment does not strictly include investigations, so try to restrict your answer to interventions.

The old adage 'drip and suck' still applies. The drip is intravenous fluid, usually crystalloid to achieve a urine output of above 30 ml/h. Many elderly patients with obstructed hernias are significantly volume depleted on admission. Adequate resuscitation reduces postoperative morbidity and mortality. The patient will need to be catheterised to measure this. The suck is nasogastric aspiration, vitally important to minimise the risk of aspiration of gastric contents at induction of anaesthesia and postoperatively.

Opiate analgesics such as pethidine are safe and effective, and should be given with an anti-emetic. They need to be given parenterally.

Extensions to station

The examiner may ask you about the causes of small-bowel obstruction in the adult.

Suggestions for further practice

Abdominal radiographs are not as commonly encountered as chest radiographs. Once again, the experts at interpreting these images are radiologists and you should ensure that at some stage you have had the benefit of a radiologist explaining interpretation of abdominal radiographs. Learning and practicing a system for presenting radiographs is essential to a competent performance in the OSCE.

Table 5.2 Common causes of small-bowel obstruction in the adult

1. Abdominal adhesions (50–60%)	The incidence of small-bowel obstruction is directly proportional to the number of laparotomies that a patient has undergone
2. Malignant tumours (20%)	Caecal carcinoma and also tumours of the small bowel including lymphoma
3. Herniae (10%)	Both inguinal and femoral hernias containing small bowel are at risk of obstruction
4. Inflammatory bowel disease (5%)	Infrequently a presenting feature of ileocaecal Crohn's disease

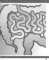

Post-operative pyrexia

GASTROINTESTINAL

Level:	**
Setting:	Structured oral with examiner
Time:	5 minutes

Task

E This 36-year-old patient with Crohn's disease had a right hemicolectomy 2 weeks ago and has been re-admitted to hospital with pain and a pyrexia. Here is the temperature chart (Figure 21). Please tell me how you would interpret the findings.

Response

The chart shows a swinging pyrexia, which peaks every 24 hours in the early hours of the morning. The temperature falls to within the normal range 4 hours after the onset of the pyrexia.

You should look at the height of the temperature and the persistence of the fever. A pyrexia after surgery is relatively common. The source of any persistent and significant infection should be identified and treated as required.

E What are the potential causes of the pyrexia?

Any postoperative complication may be directly related to the surgery itself or indirectly as a result of anaesthesia, immobility, etc. The swinging nature of the temperature tends to indicate a collection of pus rather than a generalised systemic infection, which would be more likely to present as a persistent pyrexia with no marked peaks or troughs.

- Direct complications may be caused by wound infection or deep infection at the site of surgery. These infective complications most commonly occur 5–10 days after surgery, but may be delayed as in this case.
- Indirect infective complications after surgery are related to the chest and are more common in patients with pre-existing respiratory infections. Anaesthetic gases, postoperative pain restricting abdominal and chest wall movement and difficulty with expectoration, all predispose to infection. Chest infection tends to occur in the first few days after surgery and may occur within 24 hours.

DVT and PE can cause pyrexia, but it tends to be low grade (< 38.0°C) and may be associated with leg and chest symptoms. Other common sources of sepsis are related to catheters or drains. Urinary and venous catheter sepsis can both produce clinically significant infections.

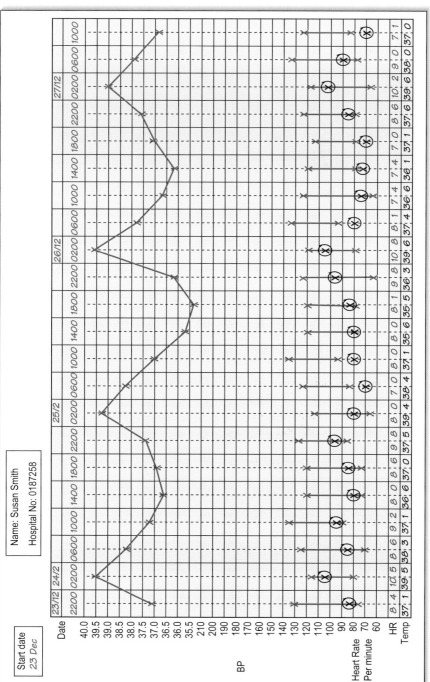

Figure 21 Temperature chart

GASTROINTESTINAL

E What would you do next?

- Inspect the abdominal wound looking for any infections in the skin or surrounding tissue
- Look for signs of inflammation around any drains, stomas, or cannulae that the patient may have
- Examine the chest and order a chest radiograph to eliminate the possibility of a post-operative pneumonia
- In the absence of any convincing source for the sepsis or any localising signs or symptoms, a standard screen for infections should be performed. These would include culture of the blood, urine, sputum and stool as well as a full blood count. C-reactive protein may rise after surgery, but persistent elevation or further increases point to on-going infection or inflammation.

As this patient has abdominal pain it suggests that the source of the sepsis is within the abdomen. Plain abdominal radiographs are of very little use and ultrasound scans and CT scans are more value in these circumstances. Ultrasound may be more difficult in post-operative patients who have abdominal pain, drains and stomas.

E The investigations have shown an abscess in the pelvis. What are the management options for the patient?

With significant sepsis, antibiotic treatment is appropriate. Broad-spectrum antibiotics covering gut organisms such as a cephalosporin and metronidazole should be given intravenously.

The old surgical 'if there is pus, let it out' still applies. There are two options to achieve this, either percutaneous drainage under imaging guidance or open drainage. Wherever possible, percutaneous drainage is preferred, as it has a lower morbidity and mortality than open drainage.

Station extensions

- What are the common causes of pelvic abscesses?

Pelvic abscesses are relatively common following abdominal surgery, but other causes include:

- perforation of a diseased viscus, including peptic ulcer perforation
- perforated appendicitis and diverticulitis
- gangrenous cholecystitis
- pancreatitis or pancreatic necrosis progressing to pancreatic abscess
- tubo-ovarian abscess.

Suggestions for further practice

There is no substitute for lots of surgical experience; get involved on the wards, day-case units, operating theatres and outpatient clinics!

Procedure skills

Introduction

As a general rule, procedure skill stations tend to be handled well by students in OSCEs. The reason for this is not clear, but it may be that students find these skills the easiest to practice and they associate OSCEs with skills. In addition, most medical schools are specific about the skills in which they expect their students to become competent. The corollary to this is that most examiners will expect a relatively good standard of performance by a student undertaking a common procedure skill in an OSCE. Surgery is a medical speciality that demands a high level of competence in procedural skills; however, almost all of these competences are learned in a postgraduate setting. There are surprisingly few surgical procedural skills that need to be learned as an undergraduate. Most of these, for example skin suturing, are considered to be important for most postgraduate doctors, but for students who will eventually become surgeons, they represent the foundations of their craft. The attainment of procedural competence is complex and not just about learning to use your hands. Undoubtedly, some people will be naturally dextrous, but this is only a small part of becoming safe when performing a procedure.

Performing procedure skills WELL

We talked in Chapter 1 about the achievement of excellence over and above achievement of competence. All procedure skills are performed on patients for a distinct purpose. Many of the techniques have been developed over many years and the equipment has been refined many times with developing technology and increased understanding of the underpinning basic and clinical sciences. Thus, before rushing off to the skills lab to 'learn' a procedural skill, an astute learner will attempt to avail themselves of all the background basic and clinical sciences behind the procedure as well as potential pitfalls and limitations. In addition, you should consider the 'people' skills involved, such as consent and communication. Although this may seem an unnecessarily long-winded way of developing a skill, it will pay dividends in the end.

Remember:

- Almost all procedural skills OSCE stations come with supplementary questions, which are based on the background information already mentioned.
- A complete understanding of the procedure will help in your development of more complex skills as a doctor.

For illustrative purposes, we will discuss urethral catheterisation as an example of how to become excellent at a procedural skill.

Urethral catheterisation

Level:	*/**
Setting:	A male pelvic mannequin and equipment table
Time:	5 minutes

E This is Mr Phillips. He is known to suffer from benign prostatic hypertrophy and he has complained of lower abdominal pain and inability to pass urine for 14 hours. Abdominal examination reveals a large distended bladder. I would like you to demonstrate how to pass a urinary catheter.

Comment

These instructions are a bit long-winded but they have been written to illustrate the clinical context in which you are likely to be required to perform a urethral catheterisation. The experience of the examiner is such that he will find it very easy to put the sterile environment into a real clinical context, as he will have performed and observed the procedure many times. Because of this he will be judging you based on this experience and will only award you high marks if you, likewise, are seen to mimic a true clinical environment.

If you are an excellent candidate, prior to appearing in the OSCE you will be aware of most of the following:

Historical background

The earliest historical records show that catheterisation was regularly used in India and Greece at the time of Hippocrates. The earliest catheters were made of metal and invariably inserted in the lithotomy position. During the middle ages, more flexible materials were introduced using flexible woods and reeds. With the development of rubber with a curved tip and the subsequent use of latex and silastic, catheterisation became less traumatic and is now accepted as a routine procedure.

Modern-day catheters are normally one of four types:

1. Regular latex/simplastic: cheap, use for most things (likely to be used for OSCEs)
2. Silastic: made from pure silicone, ideal for long term, since less infection, but more expensive
3. Teeman: tapered tip for easier insertion around prostate
4. Coudé: angled for easier insertion around prostate.

Catheters are designed in accordance with their routine usage. Note that the latter two are specialist catheters and are not routinely used.

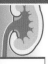
PROCEDURE 1   Urethral catheterisation

Consent and communication

Urethral catheterisation is invasive, intimate and often embarrassing for the patient. The patients are often old and frightened, and communication can be difficult because of confusion and physical infirmity, such as deafness. It follows that obtaining an appropriate consent for the procedure can be difficult and, on occasions, time consuming. A clear explanation of what you are going to do, even if the skill is to be performed and assessed on a mannequin, reveals to the examiner that you understand the issues in a clinical setting.

We recommend that you watch this procedure being performed in a clinical setting at least as often as you perform it yourself. Treat each patient with as much respect and empathy as you can muster and recognise that each individual is different in terms of their expectations and anxieties.

In this OSCE station, you may wish to begin by imagining that you are actually at an elderly patient's bedside.

S Hello Mr Phillips (extends hand). My name is Joe Smith and I'm a final-year medical student. I understand that you are having problems with passing water and I am here to see if I can help by passing a small tube into your bladder. I understand that this may be a little frightening and it may be a little uncomfortable, but I will explain to you what I am doing as we are going along. Is that OK? Is there anything you would like to ask before I start?

An introduction like this demonstrates to the examiner:

- that you have performed the procedure before
- that you have learned the procedure in a clinical setting and not just in a skills lab
- that you care about your patient
- that you understand the procedure may be painful or embarrassing
- that you understand that the patient may be anxious
- that you understand that legally you must obtain the consent of the patient.

Basic sciences

The development of the urinary catheter reflects our increasing knowledge of urinary anatomy and microbiology. An understanding of the relevance of these basic sciences to the procedure improves technique and reduces the chances of us making mistakes that can result in potentially serious complications.

Anatomy

- The male urethra consists of three parts.
- Total length is about 20 cm.

- The opening of the urethra (penile meatus) marks the beginning of the spongy urethra, which is about 15 cm long lying within the corpus spongiosum of the penis.
- The urethra then passes through the prostate for about 3 cm before becoming membranous for about 2 cm and then joins the bladder.
- The membranous urethra is the least pliable part of the urethra in normal males and contains no lubricating glands.

The relevance of these anatomical facts is illustrated in Figure 22. The insertion of a catheter will be more difficult if the penis is not held in an upright position with gentle traction. This action reduces urethral kinking and opens up the prostatic and membranous parts. Catheterisation in this position will be more likely to succeed and cause less direct painful trauma to the prostate, particularly when enlarged.

Microbiology

The three major indications for urethral catheterisation are:

- to monitor fluid balance
- to overcome a urethral obstruction
- for chronic incontinence: the neuropathic bladder.

The decision to catheterise a patient should not be taken lightly. Apart from the direct trauma to the urethra, prostate and bladder, infection is a major risk. Catheter-associated infection is a very common hospital-acquired (nosocomial) infection accounting for up to 40% of all hospital infections. It develops in about one-quarter of all patients who have an indwelling catheter for longer than 1 week.

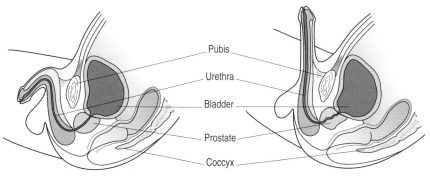

Pubis
Urethra
Bladder
Prostate
Coccyx

181

Figure 22 The position of the male urethra with the patient supine. Note on the left, with the penis in a 'flaccid' position, the urethra is kinked in two places and the prostatic and membranous urethra are tight. Whereas on the right, with the penis held upright with gentle traction, the kinks reduce, and the prostatic and membranous urethra are unfolded

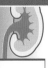
PROCEDURE 1 **Urethral catheterisation**

Box 6.1 Causes of Catheter-Induced Urinary Tract Infection	
● *E. coli*	25%
● Enterococci	15%
● *Pseudomonas aeruginosa*	10%
● *Candida* spp.	9%
● *Klebsiella* spp.	6%
● *Enterobacter* spp.	6%

Knowledge of the microbiology facilitates the treatment and prevention of catheter-induced UTI. The following reduce infection risk:

- avoid unnecessary catheterisations
- consider alternatives to urethral catheterisation (condom drainage, suprapubic catheterisation)
- use aseptic technique
- use closed drainage
- ensure dependent drainage (the collection tube should always remain below the patient's bladder).

Clinical sciences

Pathology

An understanding of the causes of urine retention facilitates catheterisation and prevents unnecessary complications. The causes of urinary retention can be divided into those that present acutely with pain and those that occur chronically, which are often painless.

Similarly, many of the complications of urinary catheterisation are easily explained by considering a combination of the clinical and basic sciences. In addition, a large number can be avoided by careful catheterisation. These include:

- The formation of strictures and false passages. Most strictures are as a result of excessive trauma. Often this is not because of over-enthusiastic pushing, but due to poor technique and a failure to understand the anatomy. It should be noted that the least pliant length of the normal urethra is its membranous part, which is not naturally lubricated. There is a tendency for the practitioner to breathe a sigh of relief when the catheter passes the prostate and to quickly push the catheter through the membranous urethra. This will cause trauma. A bit of patience at this point will allow the introduced lubricant to act
- Minor haematuria
- Hypotension and collapse (autonomic reflexes) – though rare you must be prepared for this.

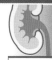

Table 6.1

Causes of urinary retention: Acute

Common	Faecal impaction	
	Post-operative	Elderly patient
		Pelvic and abdominal surgery
		Long surgery
	Spinal anaesthesia	
	Spinal cord injury	
	Drug induced	Anticholinergics
		Antidepressants
	Benign prostatic hypertrophy	
Not as common	Urethral stricture	
	Acute or chronic prostatitis	
	Blood clot in bladder	Frequently as a result of traumatic catheterisation or bladder surgery
Rare		
	Urethral rupture	Generally with major trauma

Causes of urinary retention: Chronic

Common		
	Benign prostatic hyperplasia	
	Prostatic cancer	
	Neurological damage	MS
		Diabetes
	Drugs	Anticholinergics
		Antidepressants
	Meatal stricture	Common in young boys
	Urethral stricture	

Finally the procedure!

Once you have learned the background to the procedure you need to practice. Take time on your first few attempts and as the catheter disappears down the urethra try to picture the relevant anatomy.

Core skill Urethral catheterisation

1. Introduce yourself, explain what you would like to do and obtain consent
2. Lie the patient comfortably on his back with his legs slightly separated
3. Choose a 16F* catheter and check the volume of the retaining balloon

Continued

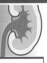

GENITOURINARY

| Core skill | Urethral catheterisation — Cont'd |

4. Open the catheterisation pack, pour antiseptic fluid into the receiver and put on gloves
5. Clean the penis thoroughly; retract the prepuce and clean around the meatus
6. Drape, so that only the penis is in the sterile field
7. Hold the penis with a gauze swab (see Figure 22)
8. Squeeze anaesthetic/lubricant jelly into the urethra and occlude it with pressure from the gauze
9. Explain that you would normally allow 5 minutes for the anaesthetic to work
10. Advance the catheter tip from its plastic sleeve and introduce it into the urethra ('no touch technique' – using the sleeve to feed the catheter will reduce the contact of your hand with the catheter and minimise contamination)**
11. Advance the catheter using a 'no touch technique' until the end-arm of the catheter is up to the meatus**
12. Check that urine is flowing from the catheter, gently using your hand to press on the suprapubic area if necessary
13. Inflate the balloon: inject the required quantity of water slowly, checking that it does not cause pain before fully inflating it
14. Attach the bag
15. Gently extend the catheter into position
16. Reposition the prepuce
17. Record the volume of urine in the bag (residual volume)
18. Obtain specimen of urine for biochemical/ microbiological analysis

---

* F = French gauge which expresses the external diameter. Each unit of F gauge is 0.33 mm so a 16 F gauge catheter has an external diameter of 5.8 mm and will pass down most adult urethras. This gauging system is confusing because it is different to the British gauge system, which is frequently used for hypodermic needle sizes. In the British system there is a range of 8–30 mm with an 8G needle being 4 mm in diameter and a 30G needle being 0.3 mm in diameter, so the smaller the gauge the larger the diameter.
** These two aspects of catheterisation are the most difficult to master and require much practice.

Station extensions

The examiner may ask you to discuss the potential acute complications of urethral catheterisation.

These are:

- infection (urethritis, cystitis, pyelonephritis)
- paraphimosis, caused by failure to reduce the foreskin after catheterisation
- creation of false passages
- urethral strictures
- urethral perforation
- bleeding.

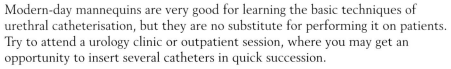

Suggestions for further practice

Modern-day mannequins are very good for learning the basic techniques of urethral catheterisation, but they are no substitute for performing it on patients. Try to attend a urology clinic or outpatient session, where you may get an opportunity to insert several catheters in quick succession.

Insertion of a chest drain

Level: ***

Setting: A chest mannequin and equipment table

Time: 10 minutes

Task

E This gentleman has recently been in a road-traffic accident. He has been resuscitated. You are the junior member of the trauma team and the team leader asks that you insert a chest drain in the left chest. Can you tell me what the indications are for such a procedure?

Comment

Until recently, this procedure may only have been examined in a postgraduate examination. Improvement in mannequin technology and the introduction of the advanced trauma life-support programme mean that many medical schools are now making it an undergraduate competency. Although this may not be the case at your medical school, an understanding of how the procedure is performed is essential and you may be asked to explain the procedure as part of a data interpretation station.

S A chest drain is usually inserted to expand a partially or completely collapsed lung. The lung may collapse spontaneously (often managed initially by aspiration) or because of fluid or gas in the pleural space following trauma. A chest drain is generally preferred over repeat needle aspiration because it allows continuous drainage and is safer as it is not inserted blindly. The specific indications are:

- pneumothorax, which may be spontaneous, traumatic, iatrogenic or pathological
- haemothorax, which may be traumatic or iatrogenic
- post surgical
- for pus or abscess
- massive pleural effusion.

186

E Show me on the mannequin how you would insert a chest drain.

Core skill	Insertion of a chest drain

1. Introduce yourself, explain what you would like to do and obtain consent
2. Check all equipment
   - Sterile gloves and gown
   - Skin antiseptic
   - Drapes (sterile)
   - Gauze swabs
   - 21G needle filled with 1% lidocaine (lignocaine)
   - Scalpel and blade
   - Suture
   - An instrument for blunt dissection (curved clamp or Spencer–Wells forceps)
   - Chest tube
   - Connecting tubing
   - Closed drainage system (including sterile water if underwater seal being used)
   - Dressing
3. Ask to see the most recent chest X-ray and check that it is labelled correctly and you are going to perform the procedure on the correct side and that a chest drain is required. Request an assistant
4. Place the patient in a supine position with the hand behind the head (see Figure 23)
5. Mark the site of insertion of the drain (usually 5th intercostal space mid-axillary line)
6. Wash hands, clean and drape the patient explaining what you are doing
7. Infiltrate the skin then move the needle more deeply into the intercostal muscles and the parietal pleura. It is not dangerous to inadvertently pass the tip of the needle through the parietal pleura. Inject 5–10 ml of local anaesthetic into the pre-marked insertion site
8. Open the end of the package containing a 10–14 French chest drain (small-bore drains are more comfortable than large-bore drains)
9. Make a 2 cm incision parallel to the rib in the pre-marked intercostals space and deepen the incision by blunt dissection using the Spencer–Wells forceps. By opening the forceps, the muscle fibres are gradually and gently split (see Figure 24). Once in the thoracic cavity, gently insert a finger to ensure there are no unexpected underlying organs. As you enter the pleural cavity you can expect some leakage of fluid and gas
10. Pass the drain (without the trochar) along the finger until it enters the cavity and push the tube into the cavity until the holes in the tube are completely within the pleural space
11. Secure the drain with a skin stitch
12. Attach the proximal end of the tube to a single-flow, underwater, drainage system

187

PROCEDURE 2   **Insertion of a chest drain**

Chest drain insertion is a difficult procedure that takes a lot of practice to perfect.

Common mistakes include:

1. Using the wrong intercostal space: it is quite easy to select an intercostal space which is too high or too low and the ribs should be carefully counted to ensure correct positioning (Figure 23)
2. Failing to look at pre-insertion X-rays: this can result in placing the drain on the wrong side, failure to notice diaphragmatic rupture and misdiagnosis of the pneumothorax itself
3. Using the trochar: these can easily damage essential intrathoracic structures. Blunt dissection of the subcutaneous tissue and muscle into the pleural cavity is essential (Figure 24). Using a Spencer–Wells clamp or similar, a path is made through the chest wall by opening the clamp to separate the muscle fibres. For a large chest drain, similar in size to the finger, this track should be explored with a finger through into the thoracic cavity to ensure there are no underlying organs that might be damaged at tube insertion
4. Failing to ask for adequate assistance or help.

Station extensions

Accurate chest drain insertion is a difficult technique that takes a significant time. Lengthy follow-up questions are unlikely in an OSCE, but you should be aware of the potential complications of chest drain insertion and you MUST be familiar with the radiological appearances of pneumothorax, haemothorax and emphysematous bullae (the most significant radiological differential diagnosis).

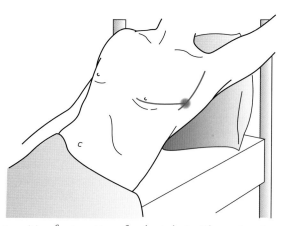

Figure 23 Patient position for insertion of a chest drain. The patient is propped up on one or two pillows with the shoulder abducted. The drain should be inserted in the fifth intercostal space in approximately the mid-axillary line

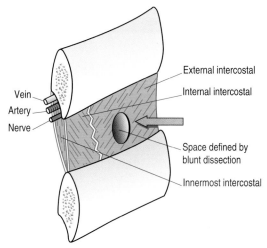

Figure 24 Anatomical structures to consider during chest drain insertion: the neurovascular bundle lies in the notch on the lower surface of the rib. Therefore, blunt dissection should occur above the lower rib in the 5th intercostal space to avoid damaging it

Further practice

The insertion of a chest drain can be stressful. A thorough understanding of the anatomy of the chest wall and its relationship to the heart, great vessels and lungs will help to alleviate this anxiety. Attendance at a thoracic operating list is very useful, because chest drains are inserted under direct vision and the anatomy of both sides of the chest wall can be visualised.

PROCEDURE 3

Managing a superficial open wound

GENERAL

Level:	***
Setting:	A latex model of simulated skin with a 5 cm linear wound. An equipment trolley including sutures, forceps, needle holder and local anaesthetic
Time:	10 minutes

Task

E This is the arm of a man who has a knife laceration on his forearm, which occurred during a street fight. Show me how you would manage this wound. Tell me what you are doing at each stage.

Comment

This type of station is frequently answered poorly because many students will focus on the technical expertise of suturing, rather than the global problem of managing a wound. This station is not designed to assess specifically the student's ability to suture, rather it seeks to assess the student's approach to general wound management. This should include a thorough inspection, examination for foreign bodies, and wound cleaning and hygiene. The suturing equipment is added to allow the more able students to demonstrate their knowledge of suturing! The bulk of marks are awarded for the student's general approach to wound management but the presence of the suturing equipment can become a significant distracter. This scenario illustrates some fundamental rules about OSCEs:

- You **must** carefully listen to what is being asked of you
- Often the skill that is being tested is not clear initially
- You should **always** have a go, to the best of your ability, to complete the task.

Managing a superficial wound

Successful management of any wound requires a careful and systematic examination prior to embarking on a treatment strategy. This station requires that you communicate with the examiner continually, so you should tell the examiner that you would want to gain as full a history of the injury as possible. You would want to know the details of the knife, was it serrated, how long was the blade and if the blade was clean or dirty. The time that the injury occurred should be ascertained because wounds that are several hours old may by severely contaminated, to the extent that they are best left to heal by secondary intention. You should not contaminate wounds any further, but complete sterility is often impossible in an Accident and Emergency setting. You should wash your hands and put on sterile gloves, if possible, to maintain as clean a field as possible and to protect you from contamination by the patient.

Inspection

You should inspect a laceration at least twice during your management of such a wound. Initially you should make a cursory inspection of the wound without touching it. During this first inspection you should assess and comment on:

1. The length of the wound (ideally measure it; this may become useful in any police or court report you may be required to make at a later date)
2. The edges of the wound. The shape and neatness of a laceration can affect the healing and scarring of a wound. Are the edges ragged? Is the shape of the wound stellate or linear?
3. The depth of the wound: Can you see the base of the wound or does the wound need to be explored further to ascertain underlying damage?
4. Are the surrounding tissues damaged or bruised?
5. Are there any neurovascular, muscular or tendon injuries? (You should suggest to the examiner that you would examine the local neuromuscular function before proceeding to suturing the wound).

Skin cleansing

Normal saline is as effective as anything for cleaning the skin with a superficial laceration. Because the wound is not yet anaesthetised, saline should be gently applied with a soft swab or plain gauze. The patient should be asked to state if he feels pain.

Anesthesia

One per cent lidocaine (lignocaine) is the most commonly used local anaesthetic for wounds in the Accident and Emergency Department because it is fast acting and anaesthesia is obtained within seconds of infiltration. The anaesthetic should be drawn up into the syringe and the smallest gauge needle available should be used. The anaesthetic should be injected sub-dermally THROUGH the edge of the wound without causing any further trauma to the epidermis. As a rule of thumb, 1 ml should be used for each 1 cm of wound. You should be familiar with the effects and pharmacology of anything you administer to a patient, so be prepared for the examiner to ask you about the side effects of lidocaine (lignocaine) and the maximum safe dose. The maximum safe dose, without epinephrine (adrenaline) is 3 mg/kg, which for a 70 kg man equates to 21 ml of 1% lidocaine (lignocaine). Infiltration should be slow to minimise the pain and the syringe should be drawn backwards before each injection to ensure that the lidocaine (lignocaine) is not going directly into a blood vessel.

Wound irrigation

The wound should be gently irrigated with normal saline. This is best achieved by squirting saline through a large syringe in an OSCE setting, although in many casualty departments a saline giving set is used.

Exploration

Using your fingertip or a cotton-bud, the wound should be probed for any foreign bodies. Gentle pressure on the wound edges, pushing them apart, will

GENERAL

expose the base of the laceration and you should carefully inspect this area to make sure there are no lacerated tendons or nerves. If nerve or tendon lacerations are present the advice of a reconstructive surgeon should be sought.

Debridement

Any foreign bodies or non-viable tissue should be removed at this point using the tips of the forceps or by rolling the cotton bud.

Wound closure

Suturing is a universal skill that most doctors require in their post-graduate practice. Moreover, it is a skill that all students will observe many times and it is incumbent upon you to ask your surgical colleagues to teach you the skill. Basic suturing technique using instrument ties is very easy to master and the authors encourage you to learn as early as you can. The goal is to approximate the margins of the wound as exactly as possible and this is usually best achieved by a single layer of simple vertical or vertical mattress interrupted stitches using a monofilament, non-absorbable stitch. The stitches should be placed as far apart as is necessary to approximate the margin and the knots should not be over-tightened.

Wound dressing

A dry, occlusive dressing should be placed over the wound.

Core skill   Management of a superficial laceration

1. Introduce yourself, gain consent for procedure and check tetanus immunisation status
2. Put on gloves
3. Inspect the wound:
   - Assess degree of tissue damage
   - Are there foreign bodies present?
   - What are the wound dimensions?
   - Is the wound complex or simple?
   - How deep is the wound?
   - Is the edge serrated or smooth?
4. Anaesthetise the wound with 1% lidocaine (lignocaine)
5. Clean the wound with saline-soaked swabs
6. Irrigate with normal saline
7. Remove any adherent foreign body: hair, dirt, etc.
8. Check suturing equipment
9. Repair the wound, usually with simple or vertical mattress interrupted sutures using a monofilament absorbable stitch
10. Dress the wound with an simple adhesive dressing
11. Arrange follow up for wound inspection at 24–48 hours and suture removal at 7–10 days (facial sutures should be removed as early as 3–4 days)

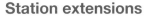

GENERAL

Station extensions

There is a lot to do in this station in 10 minutes. The examiner may ask you about your choice of anaesthetic and suture material. Lidocaine (lignocaine) is a fast-acting anaesthetic, which has low toxicity in small doses. Its effects start to wear off after 1 hour or so. Monofilament sutures are unbraided so they cause minimum tissue damage. Because they will be removed at a later stage and are not 'hidden', then stitches used for simple wound closure like this tend to be non-absorbable.

Suggestions for further practice

Accident and Emergency departments have many patients with simple lacerations. There is plenty of opportunity in A&E to observe and become involved in wound management. In theatre make it known that you are keen to learn how to stitch. The easiest way to learn is to be shown by an expert.

Communication skills

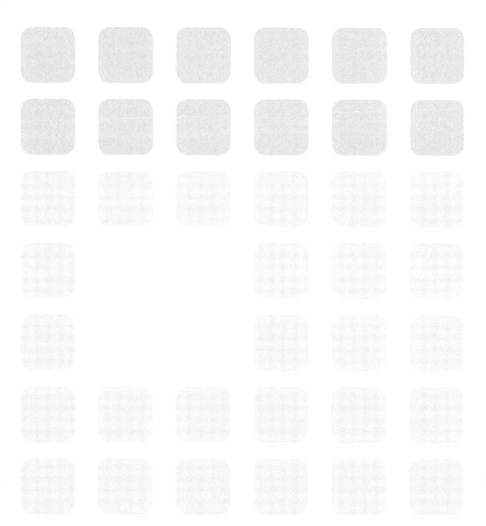

Introduction

Over 75% of the complaints investigated by the Health Service Ombudsman in the UK are related to communication, consent, staff attitudes and the handling of complaints. Of these, over 70% are upheld[1]. It is hardly surprising that all medical schools have focused heavily on communication teaching and assessment in recent years. Although this percentage may seem surprisingly high, the reasons become clearer when one looks at the daily timetable for a practising doctor.

Box 7.1 A day in the life of a house officer	
0800:	Ward round with registrar/weekend handover
0900:	Clerk three patients for surgery. Take each patient through the consent process and sign consent documentation. One patient has epilepsy another has learning difficulties. Two have partners with them
12.00:	Present cases at multi-disciplinary case conference
13:00:	Lunch with colleagues, two of whom are new
14:00:	Talk to relative about patient who has septicaemia following elective surgery
15:00:	Consent and perform urethral catheterisation on male patient (see Chapter 6, Procedure 1)
16:00:	Call anaesthetist about following day's operating list: inform them about each patient's surgery and co-morbidity
16:30:	Speak to radiologist about arranging an emergency chest X-ray for your patient with septicaemia
17:00:	Hand over patients to house officer and team on-call for the evening

It is clear from this stylised diary that the only common feature of these duties is communication and the pitfalls are many. All successful communicators obey the same basic rules about communication, whether to colleagues, patients or relatives, and regardless of the subject matter. These basic rules include:

- making sure each situation has a defined beginning, middle and end
- ensuring an appropriate setting
- using both verbal and non-verbal techniques to put the person at ease
- being honest
- listening to all that the other person says
- observing the other person's non-verbal cues
- trying to understand and empathise with the other person's emotions
- clarifying the facts using simple language

---

[1] Health Service Ombudsman Annual Report 2004 HC 703

- making appropriate time for the other person
- offering to help if it is possible
- summarise before finishing, being polite and thanking the other person for their time.

Learning to be a good communicator

All medical schools in the UK now run formal communications skills courses for undergraduate medical students. Attendance is mostly compulsory, but to develop your skills fully you must spend time with patients, relatives, medical and non-medical staff. There are many book and internet-based resources available to help you structure communication-based OSCE stations, but, ultimately, the style and skill that you develop will be up to you. One of the biggest barriers to communication-skill development is the fear that you may find yourself in a situation that you cannot handle. Many students actively avoid observing the interactions of their tutors with patients or relatives because they feel that the situation may be *embarrassing* or *uncomfortable*. It is essential that you learn to face these fears. In fact, the authors would actively encourage you to ask your tutors to attend difficult situations, such as breaking bad news, dealing with angry relatives, etc.

Many difficulties in communication arise because of a difference in perspective between the two parties. It may be that one party is less educated than the other or less gifted in communication skills themselves. Thus, although many aspects of good communication can be learned and practised, the good communicator has to be able to think on their feet and treat every situation as unique. This makes OSCE communication stations particularly difficult.

Don't lose your natural flare

One of the principal risks of formalised communications training is that the student may lose some of his or her natural ability to communicate effectively. Personality is an important part of making the other person feel at home and at ease and being too rigid in your approach to communication risks the other party perceiving you as cold or without personality. Try to avoid this if you can. Once again, practice will allow you to reveal parts of your own natural skills at appropriate times.

Communication OSCE stations

By definition, communication skills are required for every OSCE station and this chapter can not be seen in isolation from the rest of the book. However, certain surgical scenarios lend themselves to OSCE stations whose central focus is the candidate's ability to communicate. The following sections contain three different but typical examples of surgical scenarios that assess communication skills.

Explain the results of an arteriogram

Level: ***

Setting: Standardised patient sitting in an interview room with a desk

Time: 10 minutes

Task

E This is Mr Harcourt, who is 66 years old and has diabetes and peripheral vascular disease and continues to smoke. He has rest pain in his right leg and ischaemic ulcers on his foot. He is taking morphine to control the pain. You have received the following arteriogram report.

Box 7.2 X-RAY Department University Hospital of St Elsewhere

- Left femoral artery puncture, Seldinger technique
- Mild ectasia of aorta, no stenosis
- Iliac vessels normal
- Left common femoral artery. Left popliteal and trifurcation normal. Occlusion of left posterior tibial artery just above the ankle
- Right common femoral and profunda patent. Popliteal artery, posterior and anterior tibial arteries occluded

---

E I will give you a couple of minutes to read and consider the results of the arteriogram and then please explain these to Mr Harcourt.

Response

The question is about the arteriogram and how it fits with the patient's symptoms. At this stage you do not need to explain what the consequences of the result are. You do need to know the basic anatomy of the peripheral arteries and understand the pathophysiology of chronic ischaemia.

It is best to start by reminding the patient why the test was done in the first place.

S Good morning Mr Harcourt. We have now received the results of your arteriogram, the X-rays of your arteries in your legs. Do you understand why you had the test done?

P *Yes because of the pain in my legs.*

S   That's right. As you know we were concerned about the severe pain in your legs and also the ulcers.

P   *Yes.*

S   The X-ray shows that on the right side, the blood is not getting down to your foot properly because the blood vessels and the arteries, are narrowed and in some places are actually completely blocked (draws quick picture).

Comment

At this point it is ideal to pause briefly, which emphasises the importance of what you have said and gives the patient time to absorb the information. You may be wise to draw a simple diagram (Figure 25) of the lower-limb peripheral arterial system. Visualising the problem will greatly help some people grasp the nature of the disease.

S   The main problem is around the knee and below the knee in your calf. The X-ray shows that below here all the main arteries are blocked (pointing at your own knee and calf may help the patient as well as pointing to the sketch you have drawn).

P   *Oh dear that sounds bad.*

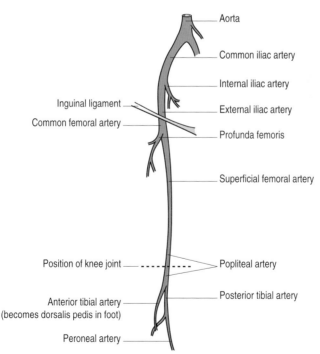

Figure 25 Diagram of low limb arterial supply. It is a valuable exercise to practice drawing your own labelled schematic diagram because it helps you memorise the important structures and being able to sketch a diagram like this for your patient will improve his/her understanding of the disease

CARDIOVASCULAR

S It explains why you have been getting such bad pain in your leg. If the arteries are blocked, there is not enough blood or oxygen getting to the tissues. This is also the reason that the ulcers are not healing, there is not enough blood getting to the skin for healing to take place. I'm afraid this means that the blood supply really is very poor.

P *Oh dear. Is it because of my diabetes?*

S Patients with diabetes do frequently get damage to their arteries. One of the problems with diabetes is that it can affect both the large and the small blood vessels in their legs and this can make treatment more difficult. We know that blocked arteries can also be caused by such things as smoking and high blood pressure. Is there anything you would like to ask me at this time?

P *No that was very helpful. Thank you.*

E I would now like you to explain to Mr Harcourt what can be done to treat him.

Response

It is clearly not appropriate to simply tell the patient that there is nothing that can be done and that he needs an amputation. Whilst that it the ultimate outcome of the explanation it is much better to get there as gently as possible.

S As I explained Mr Harcourt, you have a poor blood supply to your right leg because of the blocked arteries. Obviously what we would want to do is to try to improve the blood supply. If we don't do anything the blood supply won't get better and over time will get worse. Sometimes we can improve things with tablets and sometimes we can do operations to bypass the blockages. When we see patients like yourself who have pain and ulcers, medical treatments are not strong enough, so we do the arteriogram/X-ray of the arteries in your leg to see if it is possible to do a bypass operation.

The X-rays show that the arteries below your leg are blocked. When a bypass operation is done, there needs to be a healthy artery above the blockage and a healthy artery below the blockage. Looking at your blood vessels, because there are no healthy arteries below the blockage it would not be possible to do a bypass operation.

P *What does that mean?*

S I'm sorry to say that it means that there are no medicines, nor any bypass operations that will improve the blood supply to your foot.

P *Will it help if I stop smoking?*

S Well it always helps to stop smoking, but on its own it will not help enough to make your foot better.

P *What will happen?*

S We know from experience that pain tends to get worse rather than get better and ulcers can worsen. As you know the pain can be controlled

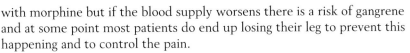

with morphine but if the blood supply worsens there is a risk of gangrene and at some point most patients do end up losing their leg to prevent this happening and to control the pain.

Would you like me to summarise what I have said to you or tell anyone?

P *No I need time to think about this. Thank you.*

Comments

The student has handled this scenario well. The use of the sketch, the clear explanation and the time given to the patient for questions and clarification are all points of good practice. There is no doubt that the patient in this scenario is likely to have understood most of what he has been told. However, no matter how careful your explanation, the message will need to be reinforced and repeated and it is essential to give the patient the opportunity to respond to the information and discuss it further if required.

Station extensions

There are many ways that this station could be extended:

- You may be given an arteriogram and asked to comment on it or even show and explain it to the patient
- You may be asked to provide advice on smoking cessation and lifestyle.

Suggestions for further practice

Giving an explanation of an intervention or treatment to a patient is a task that is likely to be required of you every working day of your medical life. Some people are naturally good at communicating a message in a way that patients understand and appreciate, but most people can learn from formal teaching and instruction on courses designed to improve communication skills. Medical schools now include communication skills teaching as a major part of their curriculum and many schools will offer additional voluntary courses and we would encourage you to attend some of these.

Informed consent

Level:	***
Setting:	Simulated patient with examiner observing
Time:	10 minutes

Written instructions

You are required to obtain written informed consent from this patient. She is Mrs Susan Black who is a 65-year-old woman who has been diagnosed with cancer of the right breast. She will be having a right mastectomy and axillary lymph node clearance in 1 week. She is aware of the diagnosis that was given to her by your consultant, Mr Jones, at clinic last week. She is also aware that she requires a mastectomy. Breast-conserving surgery would not be recommended because the tumour is 6 cm in diameter. At the end of the consultation, you must complete the consent form with the patient. You have been working on the breast ward for 3 months and are now very familiar with standard breast cancer surgery.

Comment

Informed consent is a complex subject, which can be confusing, and a potential legal minefield. Two main areas of law govern the concept of informed consent. The first is negligence, which is defined in law as a breach of the 'duty of care' that is expected of a doctor. The commonest example of this occurs when a patient develops a complication of a procedure that he/she was not warned about. This can only be considered negligent if:

- the patient was not informed about the risk of the specific complication before the procedure
- the complication is a well-recognised one that occurs relatively commonly after such a procedure (commonly is defined as a risk > 1%) or
- the complication is rare, but very serious.

The second area of law that needs to be addressed is that of assault and battery. Physical contact with any person whether it be to operate on them or to kick them is illegal unless the other person consents. The commonest reason for this law to be broken in medicine is where a surgeon informs the patient he is going to do a particular procedure and then goes on to do another.

Doctors also have an ethical responsibility to ensure that their patients are informed as much as possible before treating them. This is a complicated thing to achieve.

The student may respond:

S Hello Mrs Black, my name is Jenny Bond and I am a foundation doctor/ house officer. I have been asked by Mr Jones to come and talk to you about your operation next week. Is that OK?

P   *Yes that's fine.*

S   What I would like to do is to discuss your operation in detail, answer any questions that you may have and then, if you are happy with everything, I would like you to sign a form that is a record of what we have discussed. Is that OK?

P   *Yes that is fine.*

Comment

The student has been polite and courteous and has started well. In addition she has recognised that the consent form itself acts simply as a record of the conversation and the process of informed consent; the presence or absence of a signature does not mean that the patient has or has not given consent.

S   Do you know why you are having a mastectomy and axillary lymph node clearance?

P   *Yes I think so.*

S   Well if you tell me how you understand it and I'll try to fill in the gaps.

Comment

For there to be true informed consent the patient must understand, retain, and believe the information given. They must then be able to weigh the relevant factors to obtain a balanced view and arrive at a decision. Therefore, like in any other form of doctor–patient dialogue, an open question like this is most useful.

P   *I have a cancer in my breast that may have spread to the glands under my arm. I know that removing the breast is a fairly standard form of treatment.*

S   Yes that's correct. The cancer was diagnosed by the biopsy, which you had 2 weeks ago, and showed invasive cancer. This means that the cancer can spread to other organs and tissues, and removing the cancer can reduce the chance of this happening. Do you know why we are removing the lymph glands as well?

P   *Well I presume it's to stop the cancer spreading.*

S   Yes that's right, it may stop the cancer coming back underneath your arm but the main reason for taking the glands is that we can tell by analysing them if the cancer is already there. We need to know this information because it will help us decide if you might benefit from any other treatment such as hormone therapy or chemotherapy. Do you understand what I mean?

P   *Yes I think so. You mean if it has spread under my arm I may need chemotherapy.*

S   Yes or some other treatment.

Comment

As part of the 'defence to battery' the patient must not only be aware of the reason for having the procedure but also any alternatives that may be available.

S   When you saw Mr Jones, did he offer you any other alternatives to mastectomy?

P   *He did mention that I could have just the lump removed, but he said that the lump was quite large and there was no guarantee that he would get all of it with one operation and there would be quite a big dent in my breast.*

S   Yes that's right. Your cancer is about 6 cm in diameter and we generally prefer to do a mastectomy when lumps are over 4 cm in diameter because of the risk of local recurrence of the cancer and the cosmetic deformity. Did he mention any alternatives to removing all the glands from under your arm?

P   *Yes he said he could just remove a few glands to see if they were involved, but I then had a discussion with him about the risks of missing some cancer if I just had a few glands removed. To be honest I'm a bit of a 'belt and braces' type of person so I want it all out!*

S   OK that's fine. You do know that you do not have to have anything done if you don't want? But then the cancer is likely to get larger and spread.

P   *No I definitely want to go ahead with surgery.*

Comment

The above passage of dialogue illustrates two important points about the process of informed consent. Firstly, informed consent is a **dynamic** process that may involve numerous healthcare professionals. Mrs Black recounts her conversation with the consultant surgeon, who had started the process by informing her of her surgical options. Mrs Black is also likely to have had conversations with nurse specialists about the procedure and aftercare. Secondly, you must discuss any alternatives with the patient **including no treatment at all**.

S   What do you understand will happen to you when you come in for surgery next week?

P   *I know that my breast will be removed and the glands will be taken away from underneath my arm. I know that the operation can take an hour and a half or so. I know that I might need a drain for a few days afterwards.*

Comment

The patient is bound to have a limited idea about what their hospital stay will involve. They already have a lot to come to terms with having recently been diagnosed with cancer. One of the best ways of explaining to a patient what will happen to them is to imagine yourself in their position and take them through the episode in a verbal timeline:

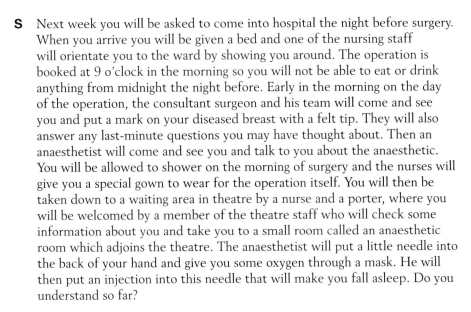

S   Next week you will be asked to come into hospital the night before surgery. When you arrive you will be given a bed and one of the nursing staff will orientate you to the ward by showing you around. The operation is booked at 9 o'clock in the morning so you will not be able to eat or drink anything from midnight the night before. Early in the morning on the day of the operation, the consultant surgeon and his team will come and see you and put a mark on your diseased breast with a felt tip. They will also answer any last-minute questions you may have thought about. Then an anaesthetist will come and see you and talk to you about the anaesthetic. You will be allowed to shower on the morning of surgery and the nurses will give you a special gown to wear for the operation itself. You will then be taken down to a waiting area in theatre by a nurse and a porter, where you will be welcomed by a member of the theatre staff who will check some information about you and take you to a small room called an anaesthetic room which adjoins the theatre. The anaesthetist will put a little needle into the back of your hand and give you some oxygen through a mask. He will then put an injection into this needle that will make you fall asleep. Do you understand so far?

P   *Yes that's all very clear.*

S   Once you are asleep you will be taken into the theatre. The surgeon will then remove your breast and glands through a cut at the front of your chest. He will put one or two small drains in your breast which will need to be removed after a few days on the ward and he will sew you up using buried stitches, which will dissolve themselves, and then put a dressing on over the wound. When you wake up this side of your chest will be flat. OK so far?

P   *Well I can't say I'm looking forward to it, but you are making it very clear.*

S   Yes it must be very difficult having to cope with all this at once! When you wake up you may experience some mild discomfort from the wound, but you will have been given some strong painkillers before you wake up. However, if you are in pain after you wake up, we will give you some more painkillers. You should be able to get up and about within 24 hours and you will be able to go home when no fluid is coming from the drains, which is usually between 3 and 7 days. I think that's about it. Do you understand everything I have told you?

P   *Yes I think so.*

S   I understand it's a lot to take in, but I will come and talk to you again when you get into hospital and I can answer any further questions for you then. As you probably know Mrs Black, there can be complications in all surgery and general anaesthetics. Do you know about any of these complications, particularly those that happen with the operation that you are going to have?

205

P   *Not really. I know that all surgery carries some risks but I understand general anaesthetics are quite safe these days.*

S Yes that's quite right, but there are still some things that can go wrong. One of the commonest in women having a mastectomy being that there is a small chance of bleeding following surgery underneath the wound. If this happens we may need to take you back to theatre and remove the blood, but this is a minor hitch and won't affect your recovery. Also you can develop an infection or abscess beneath the wound, which may need to be treated by antibiotics.

Sometimes a bit of the skin that we use to cover the chest wall where your breast has been removed may lose its blood supply and this causes the wound to break down and develop a sore. If this happens, you will need to have a dressing on whilst it heals and this may take several months.

We have already mentioned that you may have some pain after surgery, but some women will experience some discomfort in the wound for some months and years afterwards, although this is rarely severe. The glands underneath your arm are a little bit more complicated. Their main job is to drain any excess fluid that is made in your breast or arm. When they are removed the drainage is interrupted. Normally this heals in a matter of days, but sometimes the drainage does not come back properly and it can cause your arm to swell. We call this lymphoedema. Have you heard of this?

P *Well actually a friend of mine had this operation about 5 years ago and she has to wear a stocking on her arm because it swells a bit.*

S Yes. A bit of mild swelling can occur in as many as 10% of women having this operation, but severe swelling that affects the use of the arm is much rarer, less than 1%. As a precaution, after the operation, we tend to advise you to avoid injuries to that arm. If you are having blood taken, we normally recommend you have it done from the other arm. Is that OK?

P *Yes that is fine. I am sure it is more important to get rid of the cancer.*

S There is just other complication I would like to mention. There is a small nerve that helps you have sensation underneath the arm which is very often cut during surgery to your armpit. This means that when you wake up you may have a numb patch underneath your arm which may stretch down to you elbow. This will gradually get better in the months after surgery but you may be left with a small permanent numb patch.

P *Right I think I've got all of that.*

S If you want to talk to myself or to Mr Jones about the procedure further you have only to ask and we would be delighted to help. So would you like us to go ahead with surgery next week?

P *Yes definitely.*

S Is there anything further you would like to ask me at the moment?

P *No thank you.*

S In which case I would like you to read this form with me. If you are happy, I will ask you to sign it to say that you agree with us going ahead with surgery.

Comment

At this point you should go through the form with the patient. A completed form should look like this (Figure 26).

Station extensions

The examiner may ask you a number of follow-on questions. These may include:

* How may the consent differ if the patient is a Jehovah's Witness?
* What would happen if you did not know the answer to a patient's question or you were not familiar with the operation?

Suggestions for further practice

The major medical defence organisations produce booklets with guidance and help in understanding informed consent. We would recommend that you read some of these. In addition it is a useful exercise to think of the common operations that you will be expected to know about in your OSCEs and decide which information you must ensure that the patient receives and understands. This should include probabilities of the risks involved and how you would explain these to the patient.

ST Elsewhere University NHS Trust | **NHS** | **CONSENT FORM 1**

Patient agreement to investigate or treatment

Name:	Susan G Black
DOB:	23 April 1941
Hosp.	No: 07137824

Responsible health professional ___ MR DAVID JONES ___

Job Title ___ CONSULTANT SURGEON ___

Name of proposed procedure or course of treatment
(include brief explanation if term not clear)
___ RIGHT MASTECTOMY (BREAST REMOVAL) AND ___
___ AXILLARY LYMPH NODE CLEARANCE ___

Statement of Health Professional (to be completed by health professional with appropriate knowledge of proposed procedure)

I have explained the procedure to the patient. In particular I have explained:

The intended benefits ___ REMOVAL AND STAGING OF RIGHT ___
___ BREAST CANCER ___

Serious of frequently occurring risks ___ BLEEDING, INFECTION, SKIN ___
___ NECROSIS, LYMPHOEDEMA, NERVE DAMAGE ___

Any extra procedures which may become necessary during the procedure
☐ blood transfusion ☐ other procedure (please specify)

I have also discussed what the procedure is likely to involve, the benefits and risks of any available alternative treatments (including no treatment) and any particular concerns of this patient.

This procedure will involve:
☑ general and/or regional anaesthesia ☐ local anaesthesia ☐ sedation

Signed ___ J Bond ___ Date ___ 13 / 8 /2006 ___

Name (Print) ___ JENNY BOND ___ Job title ___ FOUNDATION TRAINEE ___

Statement of patient

I agree to the procedure or course of treatment described on this form

I understand that you cannot give me a guarantee that a particular person will perform the procedure. The person, however will have appropriate experience

I understand that I will have the opportunity to discuss the details of anaesthesia with an anaesthetist before the procedure, unless the urgency of my situation prevents this. (This only applies to patients having general or regional anaesthesia)

I understand that any procedure in addition to those described on this form will only be carried only if it is necessary to save my life or to prevent serious harm to my health

I am aware that cells, tissue or organs removed at operation for diagnostic and therapeutic reasons may be used for medical education, clinical audit, quality assurance or research for the benefit of future patients. I have informed the person taking this consent and list below any objections I have to such use

I have been told about additional procedures which may become necessary during my treatment. I have listed below any procedures which I do not wish to be carried out without further discussion

---

Patient's signature ___ Susan Black. ___ Date ___ 13 / 8 /2006 ___

Name (Print) ___ SUSAN BLACK ___

Figure 26 Consent form

Communicating with an anaesthetist

Level:	***
Setting:	You have been preparing at a 'rest' station, where you had been given a handout. Following this, you rotate to the next station for a discussion with the examiner
Time:	10 minutes (5 minutes preparation and 5 minutes discussion)

E I am Dr Richards and I am an anaesthetist. I am going to ask you some questions based on the handout that you were given.

Handout

You are the house officer on a gastro-intestinal surgical ward. You routinely have a 'clerking clinic' on the ward and have just 'clerked' a gentleman who is due to be operated upon in 1 week. The provisional operating list reads as follows (Box 7.3). You have taken a history from Mr. Williams and performed a full clinical examination. In addition, you have the results of some routine blood tests and an ECG: You have made the following summary notes:

Box 7.3 Operating list 27 July 2006: Start time 2 pm

Surgeon: Mr R Blenkinsop   **Anaesthetist:** Dr D Richards

Patient name	Hospital number	Age	Operation
D Williams	0156742	73	Abdomino-perineal resection

Mr Williams

Age 73:   Retired coalminer

Having AP resection next week for an ano-rectal carcinoma. Presented with bright-red rectal bleeding, sigmoidoscope revealed 3 cm polypoid lesion at ano-rectal junction. Biopsy showed adenocarcinoma, CT scan abdomen and pelvis normal.

Had right hip replacement 5 years ago. Uneventful post-operative recovery.
Gets breathless walking 100 yards on flat. No orthopnoea. No chest pain.
Myocardial infarction aged 53. Returned to work after 3 months, but on light duties.

209

Smoked 20 cigarettes a day from aged 16 until he had his heart attack.

No other significant disease on review of systems.

No known allergies. Occasional alcohol drinker–no more that 2 units per week.

On examination: Sclera a bit pale. Pulse 80 bpm regular.
Blood pressure 150/90 mmHg.
Cardiovascular system: Heart sounds normal.
Respiratory rate 14/min. Trachea central, resonant to percussion, occasional coarse crackle on auscultation.
Abdomen soft and non-tender. No masses.
CNS: Grossly normal.

Relevant blood results:

Haemoglobin	$10.0 \, g \times 10^9 \, g/l$	(normal range 13.0–17.0)
Packed cell volume	0.39 1/l	(normal range 0.40–0.54)
Mean cell volume	78 fl	(normal range 80–97)

Sodium, potassium, chloride, urea and creatinine are all within normal range.

ECG: Normal sinus rhythm rate: 78 bpm.

Discussion with Examiner

E I am Dr Richards the anaesthetist for Mr Blenkinsop's list next week. Could you tell me about the patients on the list please?

Comment

- OSCE stations with a period of preparation prior to interaction with an examiner, skill or patient are now relatively common.
- Communication with colleagues is central to delivering a high quality of care to patients.

Patients must be managed by a multi-disciplinary team that acts in unison to provide high-quality care and avoid serious medical errors. Although this might seem obvious to you, well over 90% of serious adverse incidents occurring in hospital can be attributed to poor communication between health professionals.

This is a difficult OSCE station for several reasons. Firstly, it is unclear at the outset what sort of station it is. It could be a station testing your understanding of preoperative care, it could be specifically designed to test your understanding of anaesthetics or GI surgery, it could be a pure communication station or it may be a combination of all of these things.

Developing inter-professional relationships

The interaction described in this section is potentially fraught with difficulties including:

1. The house-officer does not know the anaesthetist and therefore is unaware of his individual 'likes and dislikes'. He/she does not know how much information the anaesthetist usually wants to know.
2. The anaesthetist is considerably more experienced than the house officer. He will probably know the consultant surgeon well and be very familiar with the operative techniques used.
3. Both the house officer and the anaesthetist are busy professional people. They will be different in age, personality and temperament. These differences can easily lead to misunderstandings and disagreements.

S   Hello Dr Richards, my name is Paul Davies and I am a general surgical house officer who is working for Mr Blenkinsop.

E   That's all very well but I haven't got much time for chitchat, just get on with your job and tell me about the patients on the list.

Comment

The focus of this OSCE station should now be clear. Dr Richard's reply to your introduction was aggressive and could be considered rude. What you did not know before starting this station is that the examiner had received the following instructions:

Instructions for examiner

This is a 10-minute station (5 minutes preparation and 5 minutes dialogue), which seeks to explore the student's ability to react appropriately and professionally and impart accurate, important information to a colleague who is initially abrupt and rude to them.

You are a consultant anaesthetist who has just spent a night on call with a patient who eventually died on table following a 5-hour procedure for ruptured abdominal aortic aneurysm. A week today you have an operating list with Mr Blenkinsop, a GI surgeon, and you want to know from the house officer (the candidate) about the patients on the list. The candidate has been given the details of the only patient on the list (see above).

You should be curt and abrupt with the candidate initially and observe his response. Following this, you may begin to be more cooperative depending on how the candidate remains professional in their discussions with you.

Comment

In this scenario, the examiner has been asked to act in a role similar to that of a simulated patient. You will probably not have expected the response to your polite introduction. What would your reaction be? There are two broad possibilities:

1. S   Look I'm just doing my job. You wanted this information and I've got it. There is no need to be so rude!

or

2. S   There is only one patient on the list Dr Richards: a Mr David Williams for an abdomino-perineal resection.

Nobody likes people being aggressive or rude to them. The instinctive human reaction is response (1). In the context of professional medical practice the correct response however is (2). This is because:

    a.   You have done nothing wrong. You have been courteous and polite.
    b.   Your first priority is to your patient, who depends on you developing the best possible relationship with the other health professionals involved in their care.
    c.   Everyone has bad days. You are likely to have to work with this colleague again and by responding aggressively, the relationship is likely to become more strained.

If you consider the anaesthetists reaction to responses (1) and (2), it becomes even more obvious why (2) is the more appropriate response.

To response (1):

E   Don't get shirty with me young man. I am a busy man and I'll be as rude as I like closes the file.

Or to response (2):

E   Right tell me about Mr Williams then.

S   Mr Williams is a 73-year-old retired coalminer who has a biopsy-proven ano-rectal adenocarcinoma with no detectable metastases.

E   (interrupts)   I had already guessed as much. Does he have any problems that I should know about?

Comment

Although Dr Richards is clearly still being abrupt, his language is already less aggressive. Once again a calm, professional approach should be adopted.

S   Yes there are several things. He did have a hip replacement under general anaesthetic 5 years ago from which he made an uneventful recovery. He gets breathless when he walks for 100 yards or so.

E   (interrupts) Right. Tell me about the shortness of breath.

S He says that he is breathless after walking 100 yards on the flat, but he gets no chest pain and is not breathless at rest. His chest in resonant and there are a few scattered coarse crackles on auscultation. As I have said he is a retired miner and ex-smoker.

E So you've had lung function tests done then?

S To be honest I've only just seen him.

E Ok. Can we get them before surgery?

S Although I can't guarantee it, I am pretty sure we can and I'll get onto it straight away.

E Good.

Comment

The student's persistent politeness has led to a calming of the situation and the dialogue is now much more comfortable.

E You said there were some other things.

S He seems fine from a cardiovascular point of view, but he has an iron-deficiency anaemia presumably from his rectal bleeding.

E What's his haemoglobin?

S 10.

E Can you sort out a pre-op transfusion of three units of packed cells?

S Yes that should be no problem.

Comment

Surgical and anaesthetic teams must develop close and effective professional relationships. If they do not, the patient will receive suboptimal treatment. However, this type of stressful interaction can take place between any two health professionals. It is essential that you learn to put your natural emotional responses to rude or abrupt colleagues to one side for the benefit of your patients. When you are tired or stressed this can be particularly difficult. It is worth noting in this example that persistence in a polite attitude benefited the dialogue and the situation became less tense.

Station extensions

The examiner may come out of role at any time and ask you factual questions about his attitude such as:

- How should you handle colleagues who you think might be bullying you?
- How could his aggression be lessened?

Alternatively the examiner could ask you about the specific requirements that anaesthetists have before anaesthetising patients (see Chapter 3, History 13).

Suggestions for further practice

Observation during your clinical training is the key to understanding how to get along with colleagues. Observe the different types of interaction that take place between health professionals and look at the verbal and non-verbal styles of the participants.

Index

A

abdominal adhesions, small bowel obstruction, *173*
abdominal aortic aneurysm, 33, 82, 103
abdominal distension, 63, 172
abdominal examination, *90*, 117–126
  auscultation, 124
  inspection, 117–120
  palpation, 120–123
  patient positioning, 117–118
  percussion, 123–124
  see also specific organs
abdominal incisions, 120, *126*
abdominal pain
  history-taking, 40–49
    five-minute station, 46–49
    long station, 40–45
  interpretation skills
    abdominal radiograph, *171*, 171–173
    chest radiograph, 168–170, *169*
    endoscopic image, *161*, 161–163
  patient categories, 3
  types/nature, 45, *45*
abdominal radiographs, *171*, 171–173
abdominal ultrasound, pancreatitis, 165, *166*
ABPI (ankle/brachial pressure index), 70
abscess(es)
  pelvic, 176
  spinal, 81
acoustic reflexes, 155
aims, 2
alcohol abuse, 166, *167*
alcoholic cirrhosis, 65
altered bowel habit, 61–63
amputation, 71, 200–201
amylase, raised levels, 164
anaemia
  rectal cancer, 54–55
  upper GI bleeding, 59
anaesthesia
  communication issues, 209–214
  risk assessment, 76–78
    ASA physical status classification, 77, *77*
  superficial wound management, 191
anal fissures, 50, 51
anatomical models, 8–9
  breast, 131, *132*
  male genitalia, 107
  rectum, *92*

Angoff standard setting, 14
ankle/brachial pressure index (ABPI), 70
aortic aneurysm, abdominal, 33, 82, 103
appendicitis, 45
arterial insufficiency, lower limb *see* painful leg
  (vascular)
arterial ulcers, 101
arteriograms, *198*
  communication of results to patients,
    198–201
  peripheral lower limb, 70
ASA physical status classification, 77, *77*
ascites, percussion, 124
assault and battery, legal definition, 202
audiometry, 154
auscultation
  abdominal, 124
  painful leg (vascular) examination, 103
  skin lumps, 98

B

back examination, *91*
back pain
  causes, *80*, 80–82
    metastatic cancers, 82, *82*
    visceral, 82
  elderly people, 81–82
  history-taking, 79–83
balanitis, 108
Barrett's oesophagus, 36
basal cell carcinoma, *100*
biliary colic, 45
biliary disease, *167*
biliary obstruction, 66
biopsy
  breast lumps, 134
  small bowel, 162–163
  thyroid mass, 115
bladder distension, urethral catheterisation *see*
  urethral catheterisation
bladder fistula, 162
bleeding, upper GI, 59–60
bleeding diathesis, 60
bone metastases, 82, *82*
borderline method, standard setting, 14–15
bowel cancer, *82*
bowel habit, altered, 61–63
bowel rupture, 172

bowel sounds, 124
breast cancer, *82*
  communication issues, 202–207
  management classification, *12*
  mastectomy *see* mastectomy
  prevalence, 135
breast examination, 131–135, *133*
  anatomical models, 131, *132*
  inspection, 131–132
  palpation, 132–133
breast lumps
  biopsy, 134
  causes, *91*
  classification of causes, *12*
  examination *see* breast examination
  history-taking, 22–30
  mammography, 134
Brodie–Trendelenburg test *see* Trendelenburg
  test
bronchial carcinoma, 36, *82*
bulge test, knee examination, 149
bullae, emphysematous, 188

C

cancer
  anaemia associated, 54–55
  metastatic to bone, 82, *82*
  small bowel obstruction, *173*
  upper GI, 60
  see also specific cancers
catheterisation, urethral *see* urethral
  catheterisation
cauda equina compression, 80
chancre, *109*
chaperone use, rectal examination, 94
cheilitis, 156
chest drain insertion
  indications, 186
  procedure skills, 186–189
    anatomical considerations, 189, *189*
    common mistakes, 188
    patient positioning, 187, *188*
chest radiograph, 168–170, *169*
cholecystectomy, 166
cholecystitis, 45, 82
chronology, history-taking, 62
cirrhosis, 59, 65, 122
clinical competence *see* competence
colic, 45, *45*, 48–49
colitis, 51, 162
colonoscopy, 52
common peroneal nerve, *81*
communication skills/issues, 2, 196–214
  anaesthesia use, 209–214

arteriogram results to patient, 198–201
barriers to development, 197
basic rules, 196–197
breast cancer patients, 202–207
history-taking, 32, 36, 50
informed consent, 202–207
inter-professional relationships, 209–214
urethral catheterisation procedure, 180
co-morbidity, history-taking and, 43
competence
  definition, 8
  examination skills, judging criteria, 89–91
  path to, 4–5, *5*
  'Unique Ability,' 4
consent
  informed *see* informed consent
  mastectomy, 202–207, *208*
  urethral catheterisation procedure, 180
consultants, history-taking, 29–30
critical ischaemia, 68–69
Crohn's disease, 162–163, 174
  small bowel obstruction, *173*
cruciate ligaments, *148*, 150
cyst(s)
  sebaceous, *100*
  thyroglossal, 112

D

deafness
  causes, *155*
  examination, 152–155
deformity, orthopaedic *see* orthopaedic
  deformity
dehydration, 48
diabetes mellitus
  anaesthesia risks, 77
  peripheral vascular disease, 71, 198–201
diagnosis
  history-taking *see* history-taking
  importance, 22
diarrhoea, 61
discitis, 80–81
distended abdomen, 63, 172
distended bladder, urethral catheterisation *see*
  urethral catheterisation
diverticulitis, 45, 51
drug history, anaesthesia, assessment of fitness,
  76–77
Dupuytren's contracture, 118
dysphagia
  causes, 36, 37, 38–39
  history-taking, 34–39
    communication issues, 36
    presentation, 38–39

E

ear, *91*
    see also ENT examination
ectopic testis, 141
elderly people, back pain, 81–82
electric response audiometry, 154–155
emphysematous bullae, 188
endoscopic image, interpretation skills, *161*,
        161–163
endoscopic retrograde cholangio-
        pancreaticogram (ERCP), 66, 67
ENT examination, 152–158
    deafness, 152–155
    oral cavity, 156–158
epididymitis, *109*, 110
epispadias, 108
ERCP (endoscopic retrograde cholangio-
        pancreaticogram), 66, 67
examination skills, 86–158
    abdomen *see* abdominal examination
    breast *see* breast examination
    competence, judging criteria, 89–91
    deafness, 152–155
    ENT *see* ENT examination
    gait, 145–147
    groin lumps *see* groin lumps
    hip, 143–147, *145*
    knee, 148–151
    learning strategy, 86–91
        advanced, 88–91
        basic, 86–88
        role-play, 91, 94–96
        video camera use, 87–88
    legs (vascular arterial) *see* painful leg
        (vascular)
    legs (venous), 104–106, *105*
    lymph nodes, 98, 127–130, *128*
    male genitalia, 107–110
    neck lumps *see* neck lumps
    oral cavity, 156–158
    orthopaedic *see* orthopaedics
    rectum *see* rectal examination
    skin lumps *see* skin lumps
    stations, *87*, *90–91*
examination standardisation, 8–9, 14–15, 30
examination stations, 9, *18–19*
    see also specific stations
experience, role in history-taking, 22–25, 29–30
eye, *91*

F

feet, *91*
fever, 80–81

post-operative *see* post-operative pyrexia
fine needle aspiration cytology
    breast lumps, 134
    thyroid mass, 115
fissures, anal, 50, 51
fistula
    bladder, 162
    recto-vesical, 54
fixed flexion deformity test, 144–145
flow diagrams, 11, *12*

G

gait, 145–147
    abnormal types, *146*, 146–147
    examination, 145–147
gallbladder disease, 45
gallstones, 65, 166
ganglion, *100*
gangrene, 101, 201
Gardner's syndrome, 158
gastric cancer, 60
gastrointestinal tract, 59–60
genital herpes, *109*
genitalia, male *see* male genitalia
glandular fever (infectious mononucleosis),
        116, 130
Grave's disease, 114
groin lumps, 136–142
    causes, 10–11, 136–137, *137*
    examination, 136–142
    see also hernias
gums, examination, 157–158

H

haematemesis, 59, 60
haemorrhoids, 50, 51
haemothorax, 186, 188
hands, *90*
hearing loss *see* deafness
hepatitis, 65
hernias, 99, 119, 120
    examination, 136–141
    small bowel obstruction, 172–173, *173*
    strangulating/strangulated, 140
    types, 138, 140–141
    see also groin lumps
herpes, genital, *109*
hip(s), *90*, 143–147, *145*
    examination, 143–147, *145*
    osteoarthritis, 75–78
hip replacement surgery, 76–78
history-taking, 22–83
    abdominal pain *see* abdominal pain

history-taking (*continued*)
altered bowel habit, 61–63
back pain, 79–83
breast lumps, 22–30
chronology, 62
communication issues, 32, 36, 50
co-morbidity and, 43
consultant *vs.* student, 29–30
dysphagia *see* dysphagia
examination standards, 30
experience, role of, 22–25, 29–30
knowledge application, 33
neck lumps, 56–58, *57*
note-taking, 31
orthopaedic, 71–73
painful leg (vascular), 68–73
painful limb (orthopaedic), 73, 74–78
painless jaundice, 64–67
presentation skills, 39
rectal bleeding *see* rectal bleeding
skill development, 30–33
structuring, 32
systems review, 43–44
upper GI bleeding, 59–60
hydroceles, *109*, 136
hyperparathyroidism, 49
hyperthyroidism, 114
hypospadias, 108
hypothyroidism, 114
hypovolaemia, pancreatitis, 165

I

incisions, abdominal, 120, *126*
incontinence, 63
infection(s)
upper respiratory tract, 116
urethral catheter associated,
181–182, *182*
infectious mononucleosis (glandular fever),
116, 130
inflammatory bowel disease, 51
small bowel obstruction, *173*
informed consent, 202–207
mastectomy, 202–207, *208*
see also consent
intermittent claudication, 69
quality of life, 70
see also painful leg (vascular)
interpretation skills, 160–176
abdominal pain *see* abdominal pain
abdominal radiograph, *171*, 171–173
chest radiograph, 168–170, *169*
endoscopic image, *161*, 161–163
post-operative pyrexia, 174–176, *175*

raised serum amylase, 164–167
station format, 160
inter-professional relationships, 209–214
ischaemia
chronic, 198–201
critical, 68–69
lower limb *see* painful leg (vascular)

J

jaundice, painless *see* painless jaundice
joint replacement surgery, 76–78
joint swelling, 72

K

kidneys, palpation, 123
kidney stones, 48–49
knee(s), *90*, 148–151
anatomy, *148*
examination, 148–151
'locking,' 151
pain, 74, 150–151
knowledge
application, history-taking, 33
tested, OSCE examinations, 9–10
Kocher's incision, 120, *126*
kyphosis, 146

L

lacerations, management *see* wound
management, superficial
large bowel obstruction, 45
learning pyramid, *4*, 4–5
learning strategy, 86–91
advanced, 88–91
basic, 86–88
role-play, 91
video camera use, 87–88
leg(s)
arterial system, *199*
shortening, 143–144
vascular pain *see* painful leg (vascular)
venous examination, 104–106, *105*
venous problems, 104–106, *105*
leukoplakia, 158
lidocaine, 191, 192
limb(s)
amputation, 71, 200–201
lower *see* leg(s)
orthopaedic pain *see* painful limb (orthopaedic)
lipodermatosclerosis, 106
lipoma, 98, *100*

lips, examination, 156
liver, 122
long case examinations, 8
lordosis, 146
lower limb *see* leg(s)
lumbago, 79
   see also back pain
lung cancer, 36, *82*
lung collapse, chest drain insertion *see* chest
     drain insertion
lymphadenopathy, 57, 115–116
   causes, *58, 113,* 116, 130
   inguinal, 141
   see also neck lumps
lymph nodes, 98, *100,* 127–130, *128*
   examination, 98, 127–130, *128*
lymphoedema, 206
lymphoma, 116, 129, 130, *173*

M

magnetic resonance imaging, back pain,
     82, 83
magnetic resonance imaging
     cholangiopancreatography (MRCP), 166
male genitalia, *91,* 107–110
   common disorders, *109*
   examination, 107–110
malingering patients, 82
Mallory–Weiss tear, 60
mammography, 134
mannequin use *see* anatomical models
marking, 11–12
   'global' scheme, 12
   schedules, 11, *13*
mastectomy
   complications, 205–206
   informed consent, 202–207, *208*
McMurray test, 104, 150
melaena, 51, 59
   see also upper GI bleeding
melanoma, 98, *100*
meniscal injuries, 151
metastatic cancer, back pain, 82, *82*
MRCP (magnetic resonance imaging
     cholangiopancreatography), 166
MRI, back pain, 82, 83

N

neck, anatomy, 112
neck lumps
   causes, *58, 113*
   examination, 111–116

palpation, 112–113
   history-taking, 56–58, *57*
negligence, definition, 202
neurological deficit, 80
neurological examination, lower limbs, 103
note-taking, history stations, 31

O

Objective Structured Clinical Examinations
     (OSCE), 8–17
   assessment, reasons for, 3–4
   communication skills *see* communication
     skills/issues
   competence *see* competence
   examination skills *see* examination skills
   flow diagrams, 11, *12*
   history-taking *see* history-taking
   interpretation skills *see* interpretation skills
   knowledge tested, 9–10
   long/short case, 8
   marking *see* marking
   preparation, 15–17
   principles, 8–9, *10*
   procedure skills, 178–193
     chest drain insertion *see* chest drain
       insertion
     superficial wound management *see* wound
       management, superficial
     urethral catheterisation *see* urethral
       catheterisation
   results, reliability, 9
   simulation, 8–9
   see also anatomical models
   standardised patients, 8–9
   standard setting, 14–15, 30
   stations, 9, *18–19*
   see also specific stations
oesophageal cancer, 36, 39
oesophageal spasm, 39
oesophageal varices, 60
oesophagus, anatomy, 37
oral cancer, 157, 158
oral cavity examination, 156–158
   see also ENT examination
oral squamous cell carcinoma, 157, 158
orchitis, *109,* 110
orthopaedic clinics, 83
orthopaedic deformity, 72–73
   fixed flexion test, 144–145
orthopaedics
   examination, 141–151
     active/passive movement, 142
     hip, 143–147, *145*
     knee, 148–151

orthopaedics (*continued*)
  history-taking, 71–73
  radiographs, 71–72
osteoarthritis, 75–78, 82, 147
  knee, 151
  see also painful limb (orthopaedic)
osteoporosis, 82
otoscopy, 153

P

pain
  abdominal *see* abdominal pain
  back *see* back pain
  lower limb *see* painful leg (vascular)
  rectal, 50, 51
  visceral, 82
painful leg (vascular)
  arteriogram results, communication, 198–201
  examination skills, 101–103
    auscultation, 103
    palpation, 102–103
  history-taking, 68–73
  management, *70*
  smoking association, 69
painful limb (orthopaedic), 72
  history-taking, 74–78
painless jaundice
  causes, *65*
  history-taking, 64–67
palate, 157
palpation
  abdominal, 120–123
  breast, 132–133
  hernia, 139
  neck lumps, 112–113
  painful leg (vascular) examination, 102–103
  skin lumps, 98
pancreatic cancer, 65–67
pancreatitis, 45, 82, 164–166
  abdominal ultrasound, 165, *166*
  acute, 164–166
  causes, 166, *167*
  hypovolaemia, 165
  severity, assessment criteria, *165*
paraesthesia, cauda equina compression, 80
patellar femoral syndrome, 150
Patellar tap, knee examination, 149
patients
  malingering, 82
  positioning
    abdominal examination, 117–118
    chest drain insertion, 187
  standardised, 8–9

pelvic abscess, 176
penile cancer, 108, *109*
peptic ulcer, 59–60
  pain associated, 45
percussion
  abdominal, 123–124
  skin lumps, 98
peripheral lower limb arteriography, 70
peripheral vascular disease (PVD), 33, 69–71
  communication issues, 198–201
  limb amputation, 71, 200–201
peripheral vascular system, *90*
personality, 'type A' surgeons, 22
phimosis, 108
pleural effusion, 186
pneumaturia, 54, 162
pneumonia, 168
pneumothorax, 186, 188
post-operative pyrexia
  causes, 174
  interpretation skills, 174–176, *175*
primary care, 83
procedure skills, 178–193
  chest drain insertion *see* chest drain insertion
  superficial wound management *see* wound
    management, superficial
  urethral catheterisation *see* urethral
    catheterisation
proctoscopy, 52
prostate cancer, 79, *82*
psoriasis, 116
pure tone audiometry, 154
pyrexia, 80–81
  post-operative *see* post-operative pyrexia

Q

quadriceps femoris, 149
quality of life
  hip replacement patients, 77
  intermittent claudication, 70

R

radiographs
  abdominal, *171*, 171–173
  chest, 168–170, *169*
  orthopaedic, 71–72
  spine, 82
rectal bleeding
  history-taking, 50–55
    communication skills/issues, 50
    presentation, 53–55
    station extensions, 52
  investigations, 52

rectal cancer, 50, 51, 209–210
  anaemia associated, 54–55
rectal examination, 92–96
  chaperone use, 94
  mannequin provision, *92*
  role-play, 94–96
rectal pain, 50, 51
rectal sigmoidoscopy, 52, 54
recto-vesical fistula, 54
Reiters syndrome, 72
renal cancer, *82*
renal colic, 45
renal stones, 48–49
respiratory tract infection, upper, 116
rheumatoid arthritis, 151
Rinne's test, 153, 154, *154*
risk assessment, anaesthesia *see* anaesthesia
role-play
  examination skills, learning strategy, 91
  rectal examination, 94–96

S

salivary gland enlargement, *113*
saphena varix, 105, 136, *137*, 141
sarcoidosis, 116
scars
  abdominal, 119, 120
  legs (vascular arterial) examination, 101
sciatica, 79, 80
  see also back pain
sciatic nerve, 80, *81*
scoliosis, 146
scrotal swelling, *109*, 109–110
sebaceous cyst, *100*
short case examinations, 8
shoulder, *90*
sigmoidoscopy, 52, 54
simulation, 8–9
  see also anatomical models
skin changes, legs (vascular arterial)
  examination, 102
skin lumps
  causes, *90*
  differential diagnoses, *100*
  examination, 97–100
    auscultation, 98
    common errors, *99*
    palpation, 98
    percussion, 98
small bowel biopsy, 162–163
small bowel obstruction, 45, 172–173
  causes, 172, *173*
smegma, 108
smoking, 69

spermatocele, *109*
spinal abscess, 81
spine, radiograph, 82
spleen
  anatomy, 122
  palpation, 122–123
squamous cell carcinoma, *100*
  oral, 157, 158
stiffness, orthopaedic complaints, 72
stomas, 119, 120
  sites, *121*
  types, *126*
stroke, 33
superficial wound management *see* wound
    management, superficial
surgeons, 'type A' personality, 22
surgery, as specialty, 2–3
surgical history *see* history-taking
suturing, 190, 191–192
swallowing problems/difficulty *see* dysphagia
syphilitic chancre, *109*
systems review, history-taking, 43–44

T

tap test, 105
teeth, 157–158
tenesmus, 53, 63
testicular cancer, *109*, 110
testicular torsion, *109*
testis, ectopic, 141
Thomas test, 144–145
thyroglossal cyst, 112
thyroid cancer, *82*, 115
thyroid function tests, 114–115
thyroid mass, 112
  causes, *113*
  examination, 111, 112, 114–115
  see also neck lumps
tibial nerve, *81*
tongue, 157
tonsils, 157
Tourniquet test, 104, 105–106
Trendelenburg test, 104, 105–106, *146*
  hip stability, 146–147, *147*
tumours, malignant *see* cancer
tympanometry, 154
'type A' personality, surgeons, 22

U

ulcer(s)
  arterial, 101
  peptic, 45, 59–60

ulcerative colitis, 51, 162
ultrasonography
   pancreatitis, 165, *166*
   thyroid mass, 115
'Unique Ability,' 4
upper GI bleeding, 59–60
   history-taking, 59–60
upper GI malignancy, 60
   see also specific cancers
upper respiratory tract infection, 116
ureteric colic, 48–49
urethra, 180–181
urethral catheterisation
   complications, 181–182, *182*, 184
   indications, 181
   procedure skills, 179–185
      anatomical considerations, 180–181, *181*
      catheter types, 179
      consent and communication, 180
urethritis, 108
urinary retention, 80
   catheterisation *see* urethral catheterisation
   causes, 182, *183*
urinary strictures, 182
urinary tract infections, 181–182, *182*

V

varicocele, *109*, 110

varicose veins, 101, 104
   causes, 106
   examination, 104–106, *105*
vascular angle, legs (vascular arterial)
   examination, 102
vascular insufficiency, lower limb *see* painful
   leg (vascular)
venereal warts, *109*
venous eczema, 101
venous examination, lower limb, 104–106,
   105
video cameras, examination skills, 87–88
viral hepatitis, 65
visceral pain, 82

W

warts, venereal, *109*
Weber's test, 153, 154, *154*
wound management, superficial
   anaesthesia, 191
   inspection, 190–191
   procedure skills, 190–193
   suturing, 190, 191–92

X

x-rays *see* radiographs